LIVING WITH DIABETES

A Christian Perspective

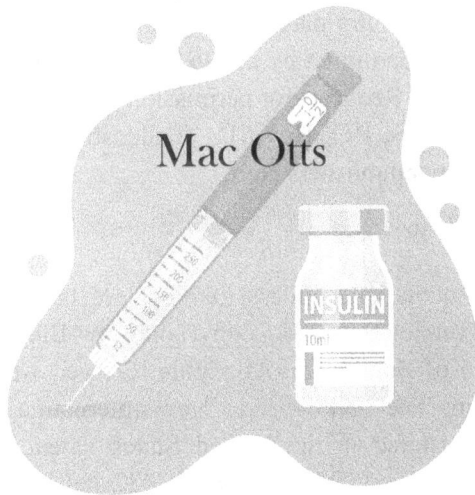

Mac Otts

Inscript

Bladensburg, Maryland

Dove Christian
Publishers

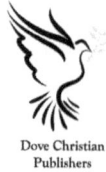

A Division of Kingdom Christian Enterprises
PO Box 611
Bladensburg, MD 20710-0611

ISBN 978-1-957497-40-2

All credit for this book is given to God, but I must acknowledge one used by him, my wife Carol, whose love and patience is an enduring contribution. God has used many content contributors, some with diabetes of both types and some with medical degrees — some knowingly and some without a clue!

Contents

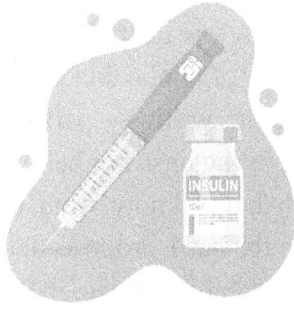

Introduction

Title Talk—Originally, my chosen title for this book was *Common Sense Diabetes*. I was writing up a storm (no small squall) when my daughter's sudden contraction of a life-threatening health condition interrupted me for five long months. Thank God, she is fine now, but a re-evaluation of life priorities took place, and I prayed regarding whether I should resume the project or end it as part of re-prioritizing my life.

I'm not saying that I heard a literal voice in reply, but there was certainly a strong feeling that I believe was Holy Spirit prompted. The project should resume, yes, but it had to be different—more open about the vital role of my faith in dealing with diabetes. The title, *Living with Diabetes—a Christian Perspective,* just came to mind way too naturally not to be supernatural!

So there I was, motoring along with this spiffy new title when I discovered that my newly renewed sense of humor could not be restrained from the writing! I added the parenthetical—hence, the whole shebang: *Living with Diabetes, A Christian Perspective (sweetened with a dash of humor).* The parenthesized part had to be omitted editorially, and that was fine since the good endorser of this book mentioned it!

Faith Talk—As an atheist and diabetic from age twelve to twenty-eight, I became a believer—a Christian diabetic. My faith has naturally been important in struggling with diabetes since becoming a Christian. Before the prolonged writing interruption, I would write and think of applicable Bible references, but they were not included in the writing—part of the process, not the product. I was hedging against nonbelievers being turned off, but hey, I'm a Christian! I know what it's like to be bugged by expressions of faith, but I propose that the often unspoken practicalities addressed herein outweigh that. While the Bible is quoted pretty liberally (New International Version—NIV), I'm not preaching down at all. This book was written by a sinner.

Qualifying Talk—From the get-go, I questioned myself: Am I qualified to write this book? I knew that there was much practical experience and common sense to share from well over half a century of diabetic living, research, and interactions with all types of diabetics. I was also confident that I could offer a different way of communicating it. However, there was still a qualifying question to answer affirmatively, or I would not have had the nerve to go for publication: Could I be transparent about my own life as a bona fide diabetic—the good, bad, and ugly? (Yes, there is good.) After prayerful self-examination, my decision was that this guy is facing the diabetic in the mirror pretty well these days and sharing it here. I hope it shows!

Disclaiming and Claiming Talk—There's four more things you should know upfront:

1. This book is full of direct suggestions. To facilitate easy review, I have underlined them. If from other sources, they will be cited and italicized but not underlined.

2. There is a lot here about diabetes, type 2, but I have never lived with it. (Most content applies directly or indirectly to both types so don't skip type 1 stuff if you're type 2 or vice-versa.) Sometimes, I dare call type 2 diabetes "little d" and type 1 "Big D". Why? It is a mystery worth solving, and you will soon know! (If that makes you feel tingly all over, you may need a little more help than you'll find here.)

3. If you are looking for advice from a master of diabetes, you

might want to just drop this book. It is about improving our ability to struggle effectively.

4. Big Time Disclaimer—I do not intend to offer medical direction (no doctor here, not even a PhD). <u>You should always run any potential medical changes by your doctor or qualified professional.</u> However, I will share medical information and advice from solid sources as cited.

I hope we both find God using the contents of this book to bless our lives and the lives of others through us. We don't have to beat ourselves up over our shortcomings or shove ourselves to improve. <u>Let's just pray for it consistently.</u>

Do not be anxious about anything, but in every situation, by prayer and petition, with thanksgiving, present your requests to God. And the peace of God, which transcends all understanding, will guard your hearts and your minds in Christ Jesus (Philippians 4:6-7).

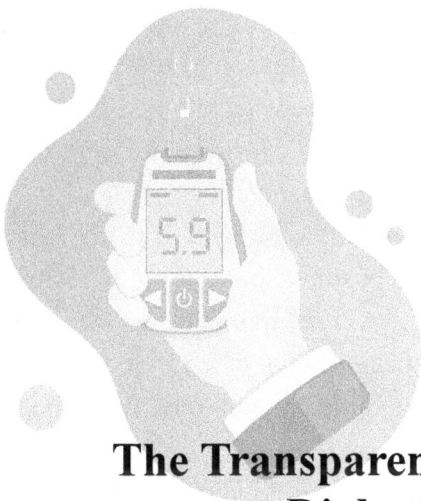

1

The Transparent, Struggling Diabetic

For you were once darkness, but now you are light in the Lord. Live as children of light (for the fruit of the light consists in all goodness, righteousness and truth) and find out what pleases the Lord (Ephesians 5:8-10).

Why such an emphasis on diabetic transparency? Well, for one thing, Christians need to walk in light—be living by truth. Besides, living truthfully is just plain good for us as diabetics. A lot of us are very capable of fooling ourselves into not living very outwardly as the genuine article—a form of denial.

After my condition was diagnosed at age twelve, I wasted a lot of years fooling myself and/or others to excess. Sometimes, I still do, but I'm facing it much better now—admitting deceptions to God and asking him and others used by him to help me overcome it. You and I are not perfect. I made a mistake once! (humor, right?) My hope is that you won't waste as much of the time God has given you on this earth as I have in denial. Denial is time wasted and diabetes untended, plain and simple.

Maybe you think you're not a diabetes denier, and the very

fact that you're still reading this is pretty good evidence that you may be right! Still, there is good reason to hear me out. For one thing, you might be like me these days—just a part-time denier. My experience tells me it's easy for us to fall into at least occasional denial for a number of reasons:

1. We look pretty normal. Well, a lot of us do. (My ears are pretty big.) Diabetes is serious business, but it is pretty reclusive. With a lot of hypo or hyper glycemic episodes, we would have to talk about it more, but in these days of continuous glucose monitors (GCM), we are better able to head those off at the pass so it shows even less.

2. We want to be normal, even though most of us, especially type 1s, have been told pretty clearly that this ain't happening.

3. We feel normal a lot—again, even more so due to advancements like the CGM.

4. We are good actors, at least most of us—if not at the start of our diabetes, then after a lot of practice.

5. We don't want to be whiners.

6. We occasionally want to spare ourselves embarrassment.

7. We may even want to impress others with our mastery of diabetes!

Many of us wear a medical wristband (bracelet) or the old neck chain with tag, but I bet the latter is more popular just because it's easier to hide. That's okay. There's nothing wrong with looking or wanting to be normal, and feeling normal as much as possible is great.

Thank God for insulin, pills, CGMs, self-discipline, pumps, and all that good stuff! Three cheers for optimism and a positive attitude! We know all too well the dark side, and maybe our noble selves don't want to burden others or talk Debbie Downer or Norman Negative talk. Nobody likes a complainer.

Okay, so a little acting might not be so bad. Therefore, we can go ahead and take a pass for numbers 1, 2, 3, 4, and 5 in the list. Still, if we aren't thoughtful about it, those things can be contributors to avoiding a lot of our problems—denial, if you will. It's a matter of balance, isn't it? Coming across as normal isn't a bad thing in and of itself. I'm just suggesting that we will do well if we <u>keep some healthy self-skepticism about how much any from 1-5 floats our boat</u>.

As for number 6, sparing ourselves embarrassment, or 7, impressing others, I don't think any excuses work, do you? Don't we know, in our hearts, that trying to hide our diabetes or faking mastery is counterproductive and just wrongheaded? Loose lips may sink ships, but too much avoidance or pride will not float our diabetic boat! <u>Let's swallow our pride, allow for a little embarrassment, and ditch the master act</u>, okay?

<u>A second reason for hearing me out on denial is that we just might see it in other diabetics and help them. Let's do that when possible</u>. It's hard to help a denier if we're in denial, at least if we are not offering resistance!

The fact that you are reading this at all indicates that you are probably a part-time denier or no denier at all (the latter pretty exceptional I think). I don't think anyone reading something like this would be a big-time denier like Fred, as depicted in this excerpt from an article by Ann Pappert, "Diabetes in Denial", published online by HealthDay:

> *Even with all the problems diabetes had caused, he still resisted looking after himself. He frequently missed doctor's appointments, and when he did show up, he parked himself in the waiting room and busied himself fabricating his blood sugar records for months back. After over 40 years as a diabetic, Fred was still in denial. His first words to me were, "I don't think I could ever wear an insulin pump, because then people would realize I have diabetes. I'm too embarrassed."*

Any one of us may not want to be embarrassed now and then, so let's don't just poo-hoo it, but Fred seriously needs help! From the same article comes this:

3

Living with Diabetes

If you've recently been diagnosed with diabetes -- or even if you've lived with it for years -- how do you know if your emotions are a part of the normal denial process or something more serious? The American Diabetes Association has a list of warning signs that suggest denial has become a problem. For example, you tell yourself that you just have a little bit of sugar in your blood, or a "touch" of diabetes. But diabetes is diabetes -- there's no such thing as just a little, whether your blood sugar is very high or just a bit above normal. Other warning signs include convincing yourself that a bite or two of a high-sugar food won't hurt, ignoring sores that won't heal, putting off seeing a doctor, ignoring meal planning, forgetting to examine your feet every day, and continuing to smoke.

You're also in denial, according to the ADA, if you don't regularly test your blood glucose levels. You may prefer to believe that you don't need to test because you can "tell" what your blood sugar is by how you feel -- a recipe for trouble. You're taking risks if you feel you can't ask your family members to change their eating habits or fear you might have to eat alone. And finally, you're in denial if you tell yourself that because you only take oral medications, your diabetes isn't serious.

Of course, even if you deal with your diabetes well, denial may creep back in once in a while. This is normal. In other cases, Laura Riggi says, fear can overwhelm diabetics and paralyze them from taking action. "And sometimes," she says, "people just get tired of all that goes into their care." When this happens, it's important that you learn to recognize the warning signs so you can get back on track.

The Transparent, Struggling Diabetic

If you're still plagued by denial, you can start to take control by writing down your care plan and health care goals and learning to understand why they are important, according to the ADA. Be realistic and remember that whatever your goal -- say, losing 50 pounds -- it might take a while for you to get there.

Remember, too, that a good support system is essential to good diabetic management.

I'm not like Fred, but occasionally, denial creeps back in. It's a tricky thing. Fooling myself and the most important people around me to the point of ignoring what is crucial to living successfully with diabetes, or not considering how my silence affects those people, or blocking out God—no way any of that's good!

We don't need to be whiners or too absorbed with our diabetes, but we do need to be open enough about our struggles to get help from God and anyone God puts in the position of being able to help us with it.

In all your travels, have you yet seen anyone wearing a tee shirt with DIABETES printed on it? I have not—same for LUNG CANCER which seems it would rate a tee shirt even more! That would be ridiculous, right? Most of us humans do not advertise our ailments, nor should we, but did you ever consider that normalcy is overrated anyway?

Everyone I know, really know, is not their Facebook persona—the image portrayed on Facebook or via social media generally—no more than they share ugly pictures of themselves at school or the office. I don't disrespect that, unless a relative or close friend is trying to project their Facebook persona at me on a personal level just because he or she has a serious condition. Here's my view: Give me a break! Please don't shut me out. I want to help you, just as I hope you want to do the same for me!

Do to others as you would have them do to you. (Luke 6:31)

To be proactive and control diabetes rather than it controlling you, reasonable transparency and the humility required for it—is a must. If this call to transparency or honesty with yourself and others bothers you, pray about it. Be honest about it before God over and over. I am confident that he will humble you as he has humbled me—over and over, right? Oh, I'm still selfish, proud, and opaque at times, but much less of all that controls me now. Thank God, I have come a long way toward letting diabetic me be diabetic me with those who care. I am trying to be an humble diabetic.

For by the grace given me I say to every one of you: Do not think of yourself more highly than you ought, but rather think of yourself with sober judgment, in accordance with the faith God has distributed to each of you. (Romans 12:3)

How confident can we afford to be about controlling all of the variables? Sadly, the truth teller must say not very, and some things are hard to nail down. A lot is unpredictable. In my experience, the world of medicine does not mention it enough, but it's still something we should recognize—the unpredictables of diabetes. In fact, I think the unpredictables are worth an entire chapter in a book like this. Consider it a coming attraction!

For me, as a diabetic at age twelve, the universe revolved around one object: me. There is always someone worse off, if not physically, in mind or heart. Every day we see them, but we don't really, really see them very much, do we? If we try to see them, we can see reality much better and respond to them, not always only to our own selfishness.

I started my lifelong journey of learning a lot more about unselfishness when I read and believed the gospel of Jesus

6

Christ. It really is never all about you if you are a Christian. I don't have to be perfect to say that. In fact, whether it is to improve my struggle with the Big D or to grow in many other ways as I get closer to the only perfect person to ever live on this earth, Jesus Christ, I have to own my weakness more and more. This has been my key in becoming a better struggler.

I want to say a little more about my faith - as prompted in prayer. My conversion occurred during a six-week hiatus between jobs. My wife was a Christian. I was not a bad guy. In fact, I guess I was relatively "good" as guys go. On the occasions when I visited church services with my faith-filled, exemplary wife, I noted something that caused me to set out to build an argument against the "inspired" nature of the book. The key was the fact that four different men wrote the gospel accounts titled after each of their names. It seemed to me that those guys may have conflicted in their accounts of the life, death, burial, and "resurrection" of Jesus Christ. In fact, I wanted to prove it!

I got a book that was a parallel rendering of Matthew, Mark, Luke, and John. It made it easy to compare them to each other, so I buckled down to study and take notes on the conflicts. What, on a cursory read, seemed conflictual, turned out to have rational reasons—so much so that I did not need to spend a lot of time on them. Instead, I became captivated by "the story" which is what I called it when a few Christians suggested that I read the New Testament in college, especially one of the four gospel accounts: "I know the story."

In college, I was always on offense, challenging the Christian faith of others. God did not exist, and Jesus was a joke. Little did I know then that the story was not as important as the man, Jesus Christ. I tried to show the story's conflicts and got shown the man! I did my best to intellectualize him away, but realized that he was everything, in my heart of hearts, I really wanted to be—too good to be a made-up story.

Yes, today, I talk and write about faith things pretty frequently, including Bible quotes, but my faith is very imperfect. Sometimes, it comes the hard way - with a lot of doubt. Sometimes, it comes when I am not feeling happy or generous or loving. Sometimes it comes when I am down, downright selfish, and even down on others. Sometimes, my faith comes after holding out for a miserable while.

Here's what I learn over and over: God can take it, but not only that. He wants it! I can talk with him as plain old me. Diabetes may affect our feelings, even moods, but God's hearing is not affected one iota. He hears me - thees and thous not required, only weakness. God gave his perfect all for me. He loves me regardless, through the point of the cross, and so I end up coming to him with thanks and joy! That's sometimes how my faith goes and ends up in places like right here!

But he said to me, My grace is sufficient for you, for my power is made perfect in weakness. (2 Corinthians 12:9)

As a Christian, I continue to learn and grow in my absorption of this principle of weakness—that by accepting my weakness, I am strong. Here is the way it was put by Paul following the quote above:

Therefore I will boast all the more gladly about my weaknesses, so that Christ's power may rest on me. That is why, for Christ's sake, I delight in weaknesses, in insults, in hardships, in persecutions, in difficulties. For when I am weak, then I am strong (2 Corinthians 12:9-10).

I understand it this way as applied to my growth in handling the daily struggle of living with the Big D: God is molding me into the person he wants me to be. Diabetes is just another tool. It has been a good one so far—actually far beyond what I could have imagined. I hope you will be encouraged as you learn more about how he could use a weakling like me. He's using me right now, and he is not through with me either. That goes for you too!

How un-alone are you and I when it comes to diabetes? Well, The International Diabetes Federation Diabetes Atlas, 2022 edition, has reported that there are 537 million of us worldwide—over 10% of the population! How about the United States? According to the Center for Disease Control, 37.3 million people have diabetes (11.3% of the population).

These statistics may not make us feel a whit better, but we sure can't assume that one of us is necessarily the only diabetic in any group, right? Even if nobody else is a diabetic, chances are pretty good that somebody is a diabetic's family member or friend. Wherever we are, somebody around us probably understands how to help if we can only manage to say "diabetic", "need sugar", point to our mouths, or just act a little weird. My experience sure backs this up. I only regret the times when I held back on sending signals.

Come to think of it, increasing positive odds is all the more reason to make sure folks around us are informed—not just for us but also for countless others we don't even know! The more informed people are, the better the odds for all of us.

For me, a tough challenge has been inviting feedback from those around me in my daily life. In recent decades, I have been more open to it from the person who knows me most, my wife of over a half century. I am blessed in that she is smarter than me and—most amazingly—has somehow managed to love me for that long. I'm not that lovable!

Whether you have someone like that or not (how many do?), bring someone in on it who cares about your lifestyle struggle. Sometimes, you can get in a group of other diabetics. I never did that, but others have told me how much they have benefitted from it. If interested, ask your doctor or helping professional about group possibilities.

Living with Diabetes

Looking back, the ideal earlier in my life would have been to combine medical professionals, a person or people who love me, and regular meetings with other diabetics where we could compare notes. If you cannot or will not do all three, maybe you can do two (like me) or, at the least, one. <u>Do not get isolated with your diabetes and infrequent visits to your doctor.</u> Diabetic self-help groups are sometimes found through hospitals, and they abound online for type 1 and 2. The Center for Disease Control and The American Diabetes Association are sources for locating such groups.

By the way, I can appreciate some criticism for being so supportive of diabetic groups when I have never participated in one. Other than feedback from participants, a reason I can vouch for it is my experience as a counselor leading self-help groups. I found that participants really invested in a group could help each other a lot more than I could as a counselor, certainly in practical, day-to-day living. Besides all they get for themselves, group members benefit from helping others. How appropriate is that for Christians?

Carry each other's burdens, and in this way you will fulfill the law of Christ (Galatians 6:2).

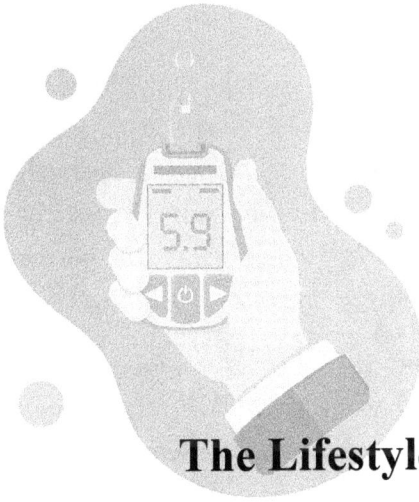

2

The Lifestyle Diabetic

You are about to have the answer to a mystery revealed. Why little d and Big D? They are different, and you should be aware of the difference so, well, so you know why I'm calling you what I'm calling you in this book—just kidding! If you don't have a sense of humor, I doubt you would have made it this far so let's move on.

We might as well get this causal thing done right here and now! Mayo Clinic is speaking here so please listen up:

Causes of preDiabetes and type 2 Diabetes

In preDiabetes — which can lead to type 2 Diabetes — and in type 2 Diabetes, your cells become resistant to the action of insulin, and your pancreas is unable to make enough insulin to overcome this resistance. Instead of moving into your cells where it's needed for energy, sugar builds up in your bloodstream.

Exactly why this happens is uncertain, although it's believed that genetic and environmental factors play a role in the development of type 2 Diabetes too. Being overweight is strongly linked to the development of type 2 Diabetes, but not everyone with type 2 is overweight.

Causes of type 1 Diabetes

The exact cause of type 1 Diabetes is unknown. What is known is that your immune system — which normally fights harmful bacteria or viruses — attacks and destroys your insulin-producing cells in the pancreas. This leaves you with little or no insulin. Instead of being transported into your cells, sugar builds up in your bloodstream.

Type 1 is thought to be caused by a combination of genetic susceptibility and environmental factors, though exactly what those factors are is still unclear. Weight is not believed to be a factor in type 1 Diabetes.

Potentially reversible Diabetes conditions include PreDiabetes and gestational Diabetes. PreDiabetes occurs when your blood sugar levels are higher than normal, but not high enough to be classified as Diabetes. And preDiabetes is often the precursor of Diabetes unless appropriate measures are taken to prevent progression. Gestational Diabetes occurs during pregnancy but may resolve after the baby is delivered.

There is actually some logic in differentiating little d and Big D so let's consider that. My friend has type 2, and I good-naturedly called him a "fake diabetic" because it is so different from the Big D. In fact, less than three decades ago, there was no such thing as "type 2 diabetes", at least not as a diagnosis. Oh, it was around before that, but doctors referred to it as "non–insulin-dependent diabetes", or "adult-onset diabetes", "borderline diabetes", or even "pre-diabetes".

As for type 1, there was no reason to number it back then at all because the number 1 had no meaning without the number 2. It was just diabetes or diabetes mellitus. You could actually say there was no type 1 before type 2! I know: This is twisted brain stuff! Anyway, I think some quotes below are pretty much straight brainy, but note that this comes from an article written over 5 years ago. Therefore, the author's 20 years is more like 25 or so years today.

As recently as 20 years ago, type 2 Diabetes wasn't observed to occur in children. In fact, it was once referred to as "adult-onset Diabetes" and type 1 Diabetes was called "juvenile Diabetes." However, more cases began appearing in children and teenagers in the past two decades due to poor eating habits, lack of exercise, and excess weight. As such, adult-onset Diabetes was renamed "type 2 Diabetes." (healthline.com)

Maybe the following quote about type 2 diabetes from the National Institute of Health (NIH) will help you appreciate the difference between type 1 and type 2:

Type 2—...Most patients with this form of Diabetes are obese, and obesity itself causes some degree of insulin resistance. Patients who are not obese by traditional weight criteria may have an increased percentage of body fat distributed predominantly in the abdominal region.

So, when diagnosed type 2 but not obese, your heft might be belly-focused, so to speak. Oh sure, I know some skinny people can be type 2. If you are one of those, maybe you should consider yourself as just a downright exceptional person! Some folks would give a fingernail and an eyebrow to be positively exceptional in some way, right? (avoiding the old arm and leg expression because that would be ridiculous) At any rate, you may enjoy seeing yourself as an exceptional person, but a warning is due: I don't advise bragging about it around other type 2s if you value life and limb (ridiculous expression too, but really common). Most type 2 folks are not as little as you, and they might not take kindly to thin braggadocio!

Both types 1 and 2 deserve planning for day-to-day living.

Even if you do need pills or the injections for type 2, there's more that you can do than pop a pill or take a shot. <u>Ask God to help you avoid victimhood and take personal responsibility for lifestyle changes.</u> He loves you, and will help you—for real. Little d or Big D, you are not a victim!

But thanks be to God! He gives us the victory through our Lord Jesus Christ (1 Corinthians 15:57).

No, in all these things we are more than conquerors through him who loved us (Romans 8:37).

For the Spirit God gave us does not make us timid, but gives us power, love and self-discipline (2 Timothy 1:7).

I really don't have anything against pills or even the more late-breaking non-insulin injections for type 2, but not at the expense of a realistic view of self and alternatives. Remember, it's easy to fool yourself. <u>Don't become more and more dependent and less likely to adopt the lifestyle changes that could help you be much more healthy in many ways, including dealing with those complications (or the more yucky term, co-morbidities) related to diabetes.</u>

<u>Take responsibility for asking your doctor or diabetes professional to help you plan how to make needed lifestyle changes, and ask that person (as well as others you trust) to hold you accountable for following through.</u>

Look, we need to face the fact that our lifestyle scores, in terms of exercise and diet, are absolutely crucial. Our society has run amuck on those scores. If you get a 5 or below on a 1—10 healthy lifestyle scale, diabetes will control you instead of vice-versa. Where's the science for those numbers? As far as I know, there's no science in it, but there is a lot of common sense!

Type 2s, please don't give in to those insulin-resistance pills or shots without exhausting alternatives, and be sure to project, with your doctor, an exit plan whenever possible!

I want us to prove those who may assume we won't do it…. wrong! Their brick wall (our brain) is our highway! Victors, right? The good news is that diabetes and death are not the same so don't roll over like you're deceased! You and I have a lot of good living to do, but a little TLC will go a long way toward making our lives worth way more than minimal living. We do not have to be perfect diabetics with perfect numbers, but we better count something! I was never a counter of carbohydrates. I do count calories, and I note the levels of sugar and carb contents.

Admittedly, it's more precise to be a carb counter than a calorie counter, but I do have a learned filter for high carbohydrate foods, and my meal choices reflect it at home and as best I can when eating out. (Wow! Is eating out a challenge or what?) My best number exercise is using a continuous glucose monitor (CGM)—easy too—reflected by adjusting on the run according to readings.

As a football fan, I like to think I'm aspiring to be the best audible-calling quarterback I can possibly be. Based on my CGM number, I just might—and often do—change my diet, exercise, and, less frequently, insulin dosage plan. It's like a football quarterback might adjust the play he called in the huddle. He does that at the line of scrimmage, calling it out loud (making it audible) when he sees how the defense aligns itself or changes players.

Feel free to use my quarterback analogy, but please do it only if you appreciate it. (Maybe you non-football fans should find something more suited to your interests—like cooking, fishing, playing penuckle, whatever!)

6.4 and 6.5 were my last A1Cs just prior to this writing. That's decent for me. Next time, it may be a little higher or lower. That's okay, but my challenge to myself is to keep A1Cs of 7 or above in my rear view mirror, and not go much south of 6. That's just my personal challenge. I am not suggesting that you adopt my challenges, but I do urge you to establish your own challenges. Some people maintain averages in the 5s, but that's tricky to me! I'm speaking of my individual situation as a type 1 diabetic, and every type 1 is not the same. Certainly, that's true of type 2s who actually have some pep left in insulin secretion that varies.

In discussing CGM usage with my type 2 friend, I found his expectations to be very different than mine. He has used a Free Style Libre CGM model for a few years, and spoke of an alarming glucose reading of his at 185, considerably lower than anything that would alarm me if it showed up on my CGM! I wouldn't like it, but there's no way it would alarm me. In fact, I have found that individual expectations may vary within types, and that's okay as long as it meets your individualized needs.

Here's the pitch I'm making: No matter what I, my friends, or anyone else does, you should set your own goals, and be sure that your qualified, trusted healthcare professional is on board with it. I feel that goals should normally be ambitious but realistic. Such decisions are highly individual matters with many variables totally in your ballpark, not mine. Don't hesitate to talk over and periodically review your goals with your doctor and/or health care professional.

Using the Dexcom G5, G6, and now G7 Continuous Glucose Monitor, I have found that concentrating on minimizing peaks and valleys in the graph is very effective for me. I keep the number 150 (an A1C of around 7) in mind, but it is not the target. My efforts are geared to something more simple. I expect variations, but I'm looking at a 24-hour graph to try to mentally draw an imaginary horizontal line across the graph as an average somewhere below that 150 figure (below a 3-month A1C of 7). Graph results in different 24-hour increments will vary above and below my imaginary target line. I don't expect to see a flat line until I flat line, and I'm not sure I'll see it then. Hey, I won't care!

By the way, while I understand the "gold standard" for monitoring glucose is still the A1C, a recently developed measurement known as the GMI (Glucose Management Indicator) is rapidly gaining traction as a way that diabetics can see averages over time themselves. It appears on my new CGM readouts, and I'm now learning more about it. While the number it shows may look like an A1C number, it is not.

We don't all have to approach this stuff the same way, but we do need to establish an approach, a method, that works for us individually. I went for many years without getting sufficient balance in this regard, and—being downright repetitious—I want to urge anyone who has type 1 or type 2 diabetes not to fool yourself. Insulin or medication alone is simply not sufficient, especially when it comes to your overall health levels in the long run. I have read that it is easier for type 2s to fool themselves, to deny their diagnosis. I have also read that more males are in denial than females, no matter the type (Fred, case in point). Both of these propositions surprise me not, and I doubt they surprise you either!

Please think about how you can reasonably work on exercise and diet in combination with insulin or other interventions to lower your levels and gain more consistency. Don't hesitate to ask for help from healthcare professionals, and, once again I say it: Try to be transparent with those around you who love you and are willing to help you be held accountable. Set goals, be real and be realistic!

Though some health professionals may not be trained or inclined toward it, a disease like diabetes calls for us to consider our lives holistically if we want to struggle with it successfully. You probably know the truth of this. Surely, you've read or heard about how overweight or obese we are overall in our society and how that has increased substantially over time—how about twenty-five plus years? Is it any wonder that type 2 diabetes got its name cranked up less than 30 years ago?

The difference between types is the difference between insulin resistance (maybe with some insulin production shortfall) being type 2 and total and permanent insulin deficiency (a total absence of insulin production) being type 1. I found the following description from Harvard Health, Harvard Medical School, to be a good way of putting this:

Type 2 diabetes occurs when your body's cells resist the normal effect of insulin, which is to drive glucose in the blood into the inside of the cells. This condition is called insulin resistance. As a result, glucose starts to build up in the blood. In people with insulin resistance, the pancreas "sees" the blood glucose level rising. The pancreas responds by making extra insulin to maintain a normal blood sugar. Over time, the body's insulin resistance gets worse. In response the pancreas makes more and more insulin. Finally, the pancreas gets "exhausted". It cannot keep up with the demand for more and more insulin. It poops out. As a result, blood glucose levels start to rise.

A number of sources say that genetics may well contribute to the problem for type 2 diabetics, but, at any rate, insulin effectiveness is being diminished environmentally. As said before, a much higher percentage of type 2 than type 1 are going to have become obese to get their condition—once limited mostly to adults but now encompassing many children in our increasingly junk-food, lazy society—just the simple truth, right? Yep, but if it's so simple, we would not need those white coated, poking people with the big degrees on their office walls. Here's another quote to confuse us just a little. It comes from healthline.com.

If you were recently diagnosed with type 2 Diabetes, understand that your condition can't eventually turn into type 1 Diabetes. However, there's a small possibility that your type 2 Diabetes is actually LADA, or type 1.5 Diabetes. This is especially true if you're a healthy weight or if you have a family history of autoimmune diseases, such as type 1 Diabetes or rheumatoid arthritis (RA). It's important to correctly diagnose LADA since you'll need to start on insulin shots early to control your condition. A misdiagnosis can be frustrating and confusing. If you have any concerns about your type 2 Diabetes diagnosis, see your doctor. The only way to properly diagnose LADA is to test for the antibodies that show an autoimmune attack on your islet cells. Your doctor may order a GAD antibody blood test to determine whether you have the condition.

First, please do not be quick to assume that you can't transition from d to D just because one source said so. Other, even more qualified, sources will weigh in on that, but what about "1.5 Diabetes" or "LADA" (Latent Autoimmune Disease of Adults)? I'm glad you asked! If you are tired of these quotes, rest easy with the fact that the following one is the last I'm copying for a while. It is from a source I obviously use when I want to impress people a lot—the Mayo Clinic! (Okay, if you are not impressed, you might be like me—not so easily impressed. So be it, but I have consistently found this to be an excellent medical resource over the years.)

Mayo says: .....Like the autoimmune disease type 1 Diabetes, LADA occurs because your pancreas stops producing adequate insulin, most likely from some "insult" that slowly damages the insulin-producing cells in the pancreas. But unlike type 1 Diabetes, with LADA, you often won't need insulin for several months up to years after you've been diagnosed.

Many researchers believe LADA, sometimes called type

1.5 Diabetes, is a subtype of type 1 Diabetes, while others do not recognize it as a distinct entity. Other researchers believe Diabetes occurs on a continuum, with LADA falling between type 1 and type 2 Diabetes.

So, apart from semantics, per the Mayo Clinic and as implied by the previous Harvard Health quote, you can indeed advance (or is it fall?) from type 2 to type 1. This occurs most likely by "insult" to your pancreas. You know, it's not as if McDonalds or Taco Bell employees are teasing or insulting your pancreas or the tiny Islet of Langerhans part of your pancreas (even though it is tiny and has a funny name). That regulates insulin for your body. Your lifestyle could be slapping your islet across the face—in a manner of speaking! It is an insult (or injury) worthy of the ultimate response—lifestyle change. I kid you not!

I don't care if it is a "subtype" or on a "continuum". I'm not a researcher, but, if it is a matter of opinion among them or just semantics, any absolute statement that type 2 will not become type 1 doesn't seem to hold up under scrutiny, at least not to me!

My Cardiologist agreed with me that most heart conditions—diabetes as well—are at least as positively affected by lifestyle changes as by medications. The refreshingly frank discussion with him motivated me to explore the same proposition with an Internist who agreed. I can tell you that getting more serious about my lifestyle adjustments has definitely had a tremendous positive effect on my diabetes as well as my CAD. The latter is not a character disorder, though I have been called a character more than once!

I have appointments with both a Cardiologist and an Internist regularly, being diagnosed with diabetes mellitus (type 1 now) at age 12 and with coronary artery disease (CAD) at age 62. As for the CAD, diabetics are at high risk for such co-morbidities (gross sounding but something you may have heard more than usual during the Covid mess). If you don't already know, ask your health professional how co-morbidities are affected by lack of diabetic control.

So the experts say insulin resistance (no matter how it got there) puts pressure on the pancreas to produce more insulin, and overworking it can insult or injure insulin-producing facilities. Over time, this means non-insulin interventions may be diminished in terms of effectiveness.

Here's what went on between my friend and me a few years before the Mayo Clinic piece was published: I told him that, if he continued the same lifestyle, he could graduate to be a "real" Diabetic (big D) like me—one whose pancreas secretes absolutely no insulin—so that he will be taking insulin via injections or pump for the rest of his life. Years ago, borderline or non-insulin-dependent diabetics (now called type 2) were to actually treat themselves by changing their lifestyles, and also possibly taking the latest pills.

If they implemented the recommended lifestyle changes and, when necessary, took the prescribed pills, they were told they could probably avoid the Big D! I believe it was and still is even possible for a number of you type 2s to actually become "normal"— meaning without any form of diabetes! I'm not applying this to any individual. Your situation may not be the same as my friend. Boo me if you want, but discuss it with your doctor anyway. Hey, you could use the term "prognosis"! It might impress your doctor! (more thoughts later on impressing your doctor).

At this point, you may think you detect a bit of sarcasm, resentment, or even anger in my view of type 2 diabetes. You may be on target about that in one sense, but hear me out before you assume that I'm just a hater. After all, my friend with type 2 still views me as a friend! I actually smiled when calling his condition fake diabetes, but there is absolutely no disrespect intended. My motivation was not to hurt him, but to stir him toward action—same here for you! I guess it's true that I hate diabetes, and I hate anything that worsens it.

Living with Diabetes

Before my friend went more radical in terms of making lifestyle changes, he was placed on insulin. Fortunately, he has since made lifestyle changes, and combined with improved medication, he has done quite well and is insulin free. I'm not by any means saying my good humored comments about his "fake" diabetes motivated him. I do know it did not reinforce something rampant in our society today, an over-reliance on meds—in my view, even to the extent of too readily including or maintaining insulin for type 2 without the off ramp! Don't forget how easy it is to fool ourselves.

For a while, my friend looked like he would be overcoming diabetes completely. That may or may not happen, but his reliance on a medication that changes his appetite levels—resulting in a weight loss of thirty-two pounds—has complicated his motivations, especially since he understands that many people coming off these medications often regain lost weight. Formerly well overweight and now quite slim, my friend has said he fears medication discontinuance. He does not want to stop this particular medication (now used by many type 2 diabetics) because he could regain the weight.

The last few paragraphs were written based on my friend's status almost a year ago. A recent discussion with him led me to request an update. I think his response, as follows, deserves consideration:

My most recent weight loss resulted from efforts to reduce the effects of tinnitus and peripheral neuropathy. I became convinced that a reduction in carb intake would help those conditions, but this assumption was proven incorrect in my case. In addition, I have known for some time that a low or no carb diet will cause you to lose weight rapidly. Unfortunately, I found that I had lost muscle as well in conjunction with the weight loss, noticing a decline in physical strength. Since the weight loss became a consolation prize rather than a cure for the two conditions I was suffering from, I gradually drifted back to some of the carbs I gave up. I have regained the 32 pounds I lost, but as a part of the increase in weight, I have gained muscle as well, a result of adding weightlifting to my exercise regime, so most of the weight regained is fat and some muscle.

I have taken a semaglutide as far back as I can remember, probably starting around 2012. I used Trulicity for some time, then switched to Ozempic because of the TV commercials. I was forced to switch to the orally ingested (and cheaper under Medicare) Rybelsus now that I am on Medicare. This drug group has never seemingly had an impact on my weight.

I am not refilling the Rybelsus now, since I have implemented a six day per week workout regime and I am beginning to limit carbs again. I am monitoring my sugars much more frequently. I may increase my once daily Glipizide dose to keep my sugars down. I have not seen the need to go back on insulin.

On further discussion, my friend said that, regardless of not attributing most weight loss to medication, his fear of regaining weight on discontinuance affected his thinking. He indicated that his initial dieting approach was a mistake that went beyond the lack of effect on the primary targets. For long-run purposes, it should have been based on reasonable portion sizes, not a cold turkey approach to carbs. Also not addressed by the initial approach was the need for adequate exercise. His new, more balanced, lifestyle approach reflects what he learned from experience.

Obviously, he has not been controlled by the fear of regaining weight, and is now on the right track for him. I hope it pays off.

Living with Diabetes

I am very concerned about the possibility of this particular fear affecting motivations for him and others. It may not be a healthy fear if it causes you to resist type 2 treatment recommendations. Please be open with your physician about it if such fear as that of my friend affects your motivations.

Hopefully, you understand that my approach to all of this is rooted in genuine concern. I really want to help stir both us type 1 and you type 2 folks to make lifestyle changes that pave the way for healthier, longer lives. God strengthens us!

I can do all this through him who gives me strength (Philippians 4:13).

Finally, be strong in the Lord and in his mighty power (Ephesians 6:10).

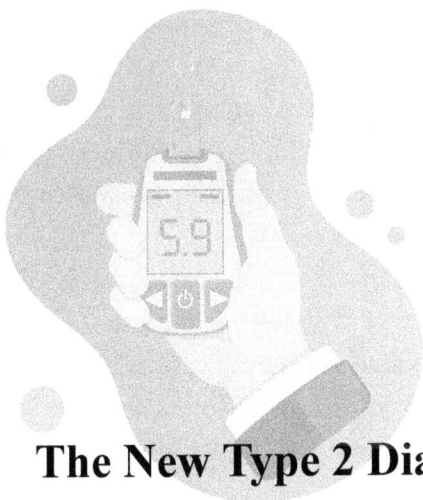

3

The New Type 2 Diabetic—A Survey

There are a lot of type 2s in this world, but you guys haven't been around that long so I'm calling you new—certainly relative to us type 1s. Yep, you are the new guys on the block! Of course, I'm just talking about the grouping as a diagnosed entity. If you have been diagnosed and living with it for twenty years, you don't see anything new about it, do you? I understand, and appreciate the fact that type 2 deserves as much attention as type 1. No matter our diabetes type, we are all the type of human beings who need help to struggle more effectively!

Still, it seems very possible that the awareness of rapidly developing resources may not have had time to catch up to the burgeoning numbers of type 2s or perhaps even catch up with those treating your condition. A more recent example could be the self-help groups mentioned before. Maybe you know about that, but who knows what you might not yet know? I don't know about you, but keeping up in this rapidly changing world is a huge challenge to me!

Since I have never had type 2 diabetes, I pumped my friend for his insights and made other efforts to better understand—research being one. Those efforts included conducting a limited survey of type 2 diabetics. The survey responses from ten individuals contained some practical reflections on a pretty personal level. I found it to be an intriguing mix that made me think of the makings of a potential ongoing self-help group.

Rather than offering an exhaustive analysis of the survey responses, I am presenting them literally as follows, copied for your own analysis and conclusions. Truth be known, you can probably analyze this stuff as well, if not better, than I can. Besides, only you know how anything does or doesn't apply to your own situation. However, I will offer some brief thoughts after you've had a chance to read the survey results.

Something I can say upfront is how different the individual respondents are from each other. Yet, I can also say that all respondents have a lot in common, and differences can be very helpful in helping each other in terms of practicality and perspective.

To explore this further in your thinking, try to imagine a conversation between these survey respondents based on their responses and how they might be able to help each other by meeting together regularly as a continuing group. In fact, go ahead and try to answer the questions for yourself. I wonder what you might contribute in the first meeting or might ask of the others.

As always, if anything in the responses or my thoughts is new to you, and you want to understand or explore it more, discuss it with your medical provider.

The respondents are anonymous to each other and to you as well. Their individual responses to each question are represented by letters. For example, all labeled A. are from the same respondent.

Type 2 Diabetes Survey—

*Note: The answers marked with an asterisk * and lettered as I. were given by someone who mistakenly answered questions intended for only type 2 diabetics. This person is currently a type 1 diabetic, but was diagnosed as a type 2 diabetic prior to becoming type 1 years later. (implication for answer to question #7?) I included this person's answers because I think they provide good food for thought—as do all!

1. What did your physician or other health professional tell you about how you became a type 2 diabetic?

A. *How I became a diabetic has never been discussed. I have a family history and have been overweight most of my adult life.*

B. *Genetics and weight. Which I already knew!*

C. *Nothing!*

D. *was told my numbers were an indication of being prediabetic. Then my A1C was taken and was told It was 6.2. I felt something about this was not ok as my sugar had always been 100. (It was 200)*

E. *My doctor said my blood sugar was too high and I was spilling sugar into my urine.*

F. *He first asked me did I have any relatives that were diabetic and at that time, I didn't know of any. He told me that most of the time it is inherited. He also told me about the pancreas not releasing enough insulin when sugar is in the blood, but much of what I learned was from me looking it up and applying it to my situation. I still don't have the answer as to why I have it when no one in my immediate family has it.*

G. *Weight gain and family genetics*

H. *Lack of exercise and being overweight.*

I. **He didn't tell me anything about why I am diabetic.*

J. *Having lived with my father who was Type 2 diabetic, I knew why I got Type 2. So Drs were telling me the new knowledge and were basically responding to my questions.*

2. How long ago were you diagnosed?

A. *20 years ago*

B. *I'm going to say 20-22 years. Not sure. I will have to look it up!*

C. 10 years or so
D. April of 2018 I was diagnosed with Pancreatic cancer following surgery in July 2018.
E. Approximately 20 years ago.
F. 15 years ago in 2008
G. 2005
H. about 13 to 14 years
I. *35 years ago 1988 (Editor note: was first probably considered prediabetic or borderline since the formal diagnosis of Type 2 did not come about until some years later, but this person did get diagnosed at some point as Type 2 and later Type 1.)
J. 30 years ago.

3. Do you take medication(s) orally and/or by injection to regulate your diabetes? If so, what?

A. Metformin, Glipizide, Actos, Ozempic
B. I take Metformin 1,000 mg in morning and evening. Have for years and has never bothered me. I take 10 mg. Of Januvia in the morning. I lost 60 lbs taking it. For a total of 100 lbs since 2003
C. took metformin but now have A1C below 7 and take no meds any more.
D. (I now take Tresiba 100 @ 22 units and Humalog with meals as needed) They started me on Metformin and I didn't tolerate it well. After my surgery, I went to an endocrinologist. She put me on insulin. Chemotherapy followed with bi-weekly steroid.
E. I take Novolog before each meal. I take Toujeo once a day I take Metformin once a day.
F. I take Metformin 500 MG twice a day and Januvia 50 MG once a day. Both are pills taken orally.
G. Yes, Metformin, Lantus, Novolog, Trulicity
H. I take Metformin twice a day, no injections.

I.   *Novolog

J.   Yes, Lantus by injection and Januvia by pill.

4. What are the most important lessons you have learned about regulating it?

A.   Limit carbs and exercise regularly.

B.   You have to find out which foods make it go up! And exercise. Best to keep a daily chart of what you eat, til you see what causes your sugar to go up!

C.   take care with what you eat.

D.   Carbohydrates come in different forms. READ LABELS

E.   I need to cut down on my portions of meals.

F.   Low carb foods in the diet are as important as low sugar intake. Also, when my sugar is high, I drink lots of water and exercise, if it's nothing more than a walk down the street. But staying on a regular exercise routine is important in keeping it down.

G.   Proper diet – low carbs, zero sugars

H.   Mine has always been under very good control, I have only once or twice had an A1C over 7. I am still technically prediabetic most of the time with reading around 6.5 - 6.7. I don't have to check my sugar daily, just every so often to keep track of what it is reading. Unfortunately, because of that, it has not been a major factor in my everyday life. As I get older, I am starting to think more about addressing it with food choices and weight loss.

I.   *Taking my insulin at the right time and checking my blood with my meter at least 4 times a day.

J.   #1 After 30 years on Metformin and Glyburide, my renal doctor, having diagnosed Stage 4 renal disease, told me those two medicines cause Kidney Disease!!!!! What the heck... why are so many diabetics who will have kidney disease continue to be put on these meds. Pharmaceutical companies are so immoral. #2. Do what ever it takes to *reduce food intake. I have a lap band and it has controlled my weight for last 15 years.*

5. Is there anything about type 2 that has surprised you after you were diagnosed and lived with it a while?

A. *How rapidly I lost weight after going off insulin.*

B. *Thankful that I wasn't as severe a diabetic as my mama was!*

C. *no*

D. *For me, I think it was the first sign of the pancreatic cancer*

E. *I have been surprised at the high and low spikes in blood sugar with no viable reasoning.*

F. *Oh my! All the things that are caused by diabetes, from heart trouble on down to ingrown toenails.*

G. *No*

H. *It really is a very silent disease for me. It has not made a big difference in my lifestyle. I know that can and will probably change.*

I. **Surprise about how fast my numbers change after eating.*

J. *No... It was a small burden to bear, but did not prevent me from doing all things I wanted to do.*

6. What is your toughest challenge when it comes to regulating your diabetes?

A. *Avoiding sweets and snacks.*

B. *Getting the munchies!*

C. *limiting sweets*

D. *Eating the right balance of foods*

E. *Regulating portions and types of food. It is a nightmare trying to find healthy food when eating out.*

F. *Staying on the low carb diet is tough. No bread, potatoes and many vegetables. I can handle the no sugar. It's just hard not to be able to eat the things you love. A big challenge for me is eating at functions where you don't have a choice of the menu. Many times they serve high carb foods, vegetables with added sugar and a nice big sugary dessert. Many times I have gone home hungry and had to eat when I got home.*

G. *Diet (I am a carb craver)*

H. *planning meals and weight loss and exercise*

I. **Knowing what foods affects my numbers and giving up pecan pie.*

J. *Eating less cookies, candies, and chips.*

7. Do you think your type 2 could ever become type 1?

A. *I believe as long as I am in good control it will not happen.*

B. *No! Sometimes I think my pancreas does work!*

C. *no idea*

D. *40% of my pancreas was removed during the Whipple. Each CT says the pancreas shows signs of atrophy. One doctor said I was not a true type 2!*

E. *I have no idea.*

F. *I don't know about that. I have heard that many type 2 have ended up on insulin with uncontrolled diabetes but have never heard of any type 2 becoming type 1. I am pretty good with keeping it controlled.*

G. *No*

H. *No, so far it is under very good control.*

I. **Yes*

J. *No, it is not possible.*

8. Is there anything you would like your doctor or health professional to do differently in helping you regulate your diabetes? If so, what?

A. *I am 100% satisfied with my doctor.*

B. *No!*

C. *no*

D. *no*

E. *Not being a doctor, I have no choice but to trust them.*

F. *I have already confronted my physician about changing my medication. When things are going good he switches me to something else or reduces the dosage, my sugar goes out of control. I told him "if it ain't broke, don't fix it." Also, I wish he would quit telling me that I'm doing good. As long as My A1C is under 7, that is under the guidelines. That is not incentive for me to do better. I am still developing problems from diabetes. I would rather him tell me to keep working to make it better so that I won't develop problems.*

G. *No*

H. *I want medication that contributes to weight loss also.*

I. **More information about diabetes. Classes on managing and controlling diabetes.*

J. *I wish I had one Doctor of Diabetes instead of having an Internal Medicine Dr., a Podiatrist, a Renal Dr., a Urogynocologist, a cardiologist etc.*

9. Is your diabetes ever awkward or embarrassing for you? If so, please explain.

A. *No.*

B. *No!*

C. *no*

D. *___*

E. *Some times when eating out with friends and my blood sugar is high, I pass on eating all together*

F. *Yes of course. When I am at a restaurant or eating with a group of friends and have to take a pill or check my sugar to see if you can eat what's served. It's also embarrassing to me when people think you are diabetic because you eat too much or you are fat.*

G. *No*

H. *No, not so far*

I. **No it's part of who I am.*

J. *No. God will help me face each day and will allow me to be proud, not embarrassed by this condition He chose for me.*

10. Rate yourself on a 1 to 10 scale as to making good life-style adjustments (diet, exercise) to regulate your diabetes, with 1 being the worst and 10 the best you could possibly do.

A. *At this point I would rate myself a 9.*

B. *Probably a 6. I could do better. Exercise. But bad knees and hips. Fixing to take care of one knee and (my area) just got a Gym and found out today they have signed up with Silver Sneakers. So I'm going to do that!*

C. *7-8*

D. *I rate myself an 8. I am always trying to be more active and make better food choices too.*

E. *5*

F. *I do believe I am a 8 taking in to consideration that it's the best I can do.*

G. *8*

H. *I rate myself a 5, I am not the worst, but definitely not doing my best. My doctor tells me that if I get really serious about exercising and lose just 20 or 30 pounds, I could maybe cut my medication or come off completely. So, like I said, I haven't always taken my diabetes very seriously, but as I age, I am starting to think more about my longevity and how it might affect that.*

I. **9*

J. *I have occasional bouts of depression... not always Diabetes caused, but in general, I think I would be about an 8.*

Thoughts on responses - These are for you to ponder or toss in the thought garbage bin:

First, I must say that I may or may not agree with statements of opinion made by survey respondents. Doctors did not discuss causes very often. Why might that matter or not? There were no diabetic rookies in this group. What might it mean to a rookie to get in on a veteran discussion? The variety of medications is amazing. Do you know why yours is especially suited to your needs? I noted that 4 of the 9 current type 2s are on some form of insulin but not necessarily insulin alone.

Lessons learned are pretty heavy (no pun intended) on sugar, carbs, and exercise—just saying. Surprises for respondents include weight loss, glucose unpredictability, and related complications. The greatest challenges they named are very consistent in terms of diet, but only one mentioned exercise. I had no idea the survey was answered by so many dedicated fitness folks! (just joking or lol)

As for number 7, could type 2s graduate (maybe better said, devolve) into type 1s? I have found this to be a bit conflictual and perhaps not entirely resolved for many diabetics, but what about research and treating professionals? Maybe it's above my pay grade, but there's more on this herein. (Don't forget the asterisk* answer on this!) On what you'd like from your doctor, we trust them, or we shouldn't have them, right? Still, we are consumers, and they will admit imperfection (if not, move on quickly) so ....

Only two respondents confessed to any embarrassment or awkwardness. Count me in with them. Do any of the others take injections prior to meals when eating out? (That's the socially sensitive type 1 in me talking.) The self-rating scores average about a C+. It only means something if you have room for improvement, and are able to be objective. I'm giving myself an 8. (I am not one bit surprised that there's no 10s, but should a 9 be writing this book?)

The Bible has a lot to say about helping each other. We shouldn't just consider what we can gain to help us manage our diabetes successfully. You and I should also think about how we may be able to help others manage their diabetes. Small groups are one way we can do that. You don't have to be a big talker or even a good talker. In fact, I'm not convinced that good talkers help folks any more than good listeners! (If you are a good talker,

I mean no offense!) Including our faith, don't you agree that the most important thing we can offer each other is caring?

> **Jesus replied: "'Love the Lord your God with all your heart and with all your soul and with all your mind.' This is the first and greatest commandment. And the second is like it: 'Love your neighbor as yourself'" (Matthew 22:37-39).**

4

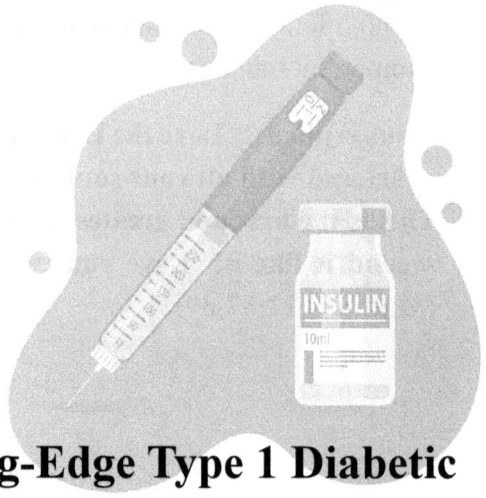

The Cutting-Edge Type 1 Diabetic

I don't know about you, but I am definitely not on the "cutting edge" as a diabetic. What I mean is that I don't claim to be up to speed on using the latest technology or staying fully informed on day-to-day research findings. Hopefully, this chapter will be helpful for you and me as we get just a little sharper, but I don't think I will ever be able to claim to be a cutting-edge diabetic, and that's okay. However, the good news is that I know one! I will use him as a resource, and I will offer some research as well.

If you are type 1, you might even say I'm a "dull edge" diabetic, depending on how close you are to the edge! I am using the Dexcom 7 Continuous Glucose Monitor at the time of this writing, can share a lot about that, and it certainly relates to other CGM systems. First, here's the Mayo Clinic's definition of a few things in case you need a little primer for something that will be considered by my cutting-edge friend.

An insulin pump is a small, computerized device worn outside of the body that delivers insulin under the skin. A hybrid closed loop insulin pump attempts to mimic the body's natural communication loop by linking with a secondary device called a continuous glucose monitor, or CGM, sensor and automatically adjusting some of the insulin delivered based on continually monitored blood sugar levels.

The term "hybrid" is used because it is not a full closed loop. Although the system can monitor blood sugars and adjust insulin based on the data, it needs to be adjusted manually when a person eats a meal or if there is a sudden rise in blood sugar. It has been approved for use by people with Type 1 and Type 2 diabetes.

I do not use an insulin pump. At first, my reject reasoning was almost Fredish (new word—remember Fred?). I did not want a mechanism attached to my body and had maintenance and replacement insecurities regarding the pump. At the time, I still fancied myself a competitive, decent athlete. I did not think the pump would help. I thought it might even hinder me, and would not look good. Not that I looked so good anyway, but there was hair on my head then!

Some years later, all of that mattered to me much less, but I had another concern about the pump that became bigger to me as I began to entertain another potential device, the continuous glucose monitor (CGM). I did not want to deal with maintenance and replacement issues in order to avoid the inconvenience of injecting myself—even though socially and circumstantially challenging, not to mention pain and occasional atrophy!

On the other hand, I was sold on the CGM, and it overrode any maintenance/replacement concerns very quickly for two pretty good reasons: First, I would much rather avoid finger pricks than shots! Extremities simply hurt more, at least to me. Second, I could be anywhere, anytime, and know that all-important glucose score!

There's more to think about beyond the revolutionary CGM. When I first considered this chapter on the cutting-edge diabetic, somebody automatically came to mind. He is a good bit younger than me, a lot smarter, and I just knew he would be the true cutting-edge diabetic! He's a chief Chemical Engineer whose work entails pharmaceutical research/development and an awareness of how the rubber meets the road in medical-related developments.

The reason this individual immediately came to mind relates to an exchange we had a long time ago. As a type 1 diabetic and after experience in personally using an insulin pump, he was invited (by way of his friend, my son) to try to persuade dull-edge yours truly to use one. He enthusiastically took on this sharpening challenge, did not convert me to the pump, but I was totally impressed with his presentation and ability to field my sometimes goofy but ranging questions. Today, this man works on the pharmaceutical cutting edge. I felt that he was probably up to speed on new and prospective developments. So, to make a medium size story real short, I went to him. He did not disappoint.

For purposes of this chapter, I will refer to this cutting-edge diabetic as CE. My reasoning for using this moniker is twofold: 1. I requested transparency, and his job is sensitive. 2. CE not only stands for Cutting Edge, but for Chemical Engineer too! Following are some questions I posed and CE's answers. He currently uses both the insulin pump and the CGM but not a closed-loop system—yet.

1. Please discuss how your background has prepared you to talk about diabetes on the "cutting edge."

CE: *I was diagnosed with diabetes at 10 years old. I used daily insulin injections (twice a day for a few years, then thrice a day) until about the year 2000 when I began using an insulin pump while in college. The pump allowed much better BG control and much more flexibility in my schedule and lifestyle, especially while running cross country and track. I first tried a ... continuous glucose monitor in the early 2000s, but I stopped after a short time for multiple reasons (introducer "harpoon" so large, significant inaccuracies in BG readings compared to finger stick). I then started using the Dexcom G5 sensor in the mid-2010s and moved to the Dexcom G6 in around 2018. The CGM again made life much more flexible and allowed better BG control. Eliminating the need for finger stick calibrations has made the G6 a great help. I continue to live an active lifestyle and use my pump and CGM to manage my diabetes.*

2. What pluses and minuses do you see for using any current version of a closed loop system?

CE: *Pluses - Easier BG control is certainly an advantage for closed loop control. I won't say "better" control since I have known people who controlled their A1C below 6 without the use of an insulin pump or CGM - but it seems to be much less work. I am considering switching to a new pump and will likely start using a closed-loop system at that time.*

Minuses - My current pump...is not compatible with my CGM... for closed-loop control. Additionally, I have a bit of reluctance to go to closed-loop since there are sometimes inaccuracies with CGM sensors as well as delivery problems with the insulin pump (damaged/leaking infusion set, scar tissue, etc.)

3. What progressive future developments along these lines, or toward an "artificial pancreas," do you anticipate and how soon do you think such developments may realistically be available?

CE: *I had heard of potential development of CGM systems that directly monitor blood, but I'm not sure I would want to have a surgical implant for such a device. Same goes for an implanted insulin pump or delivery device. I think technology improvements and new devices to help manage diabetes are great! However, I am reluctant to become too dependent on devices, particularly for closed-loop control where the devices may be controlling based on inaccurate data.*

4. As a diabetic on the cutting edge, what other developing interventions or cure potentials do you believe hold the greatest promise? Please say anything about them that you regard as important.

CE: *Gene therapies seem to hold the greatest promise right now for eliminating Type 1 diabetes. I seem to remember even implanting donor islet cells/beta cells to restart insulin production had issues, but "reprogramming" the body's own pancreas to begin producing insulin again would be wonderful. I recently read that two diabetic patients received stem cell treatments, and after one infusion, both experienced restored insulin production and blood glucose levels.*

I think it is not so much a question of what is possible, but what will actually be brought to market and how the diabetes care industry would adapt to having a bona fide "cure." This new paradigm is already being tested for a number of serious rare diseases, but such a paradigm shift for Type 1 diabetes would seemingly be much more impactful to the marketplace. I am certainly not "anti-big pharma" since I have been an engineer in the pharma industry for around 20 years, but I think there would be - and probably should be - a major shift in the pharma and medical device industry in response to such an advent.

I found CE's responses to be both optimistic and realistic— certainly transparent. I definitely thought that the elusive cure for diabetes might not be on the horizon anytime soon, but something similar to an artificial pancreas might not be so distant. Still, a number of experienced diabetics I have spoken to remain unconvinced regarding use of existing closed-loop systems. Then, CE subsequently added this comment that caused me to do a double-take:

CE: *Just to add to this, there is also the Tandem t:slim insulin pump that is compatible with the Dexcom G6 CGM (this is the pump I am considering). Additionally, there is the Beta Bionics iLet "bionic pancreas" that uses Dexcom CGM readings and does not require entry of basal rates, carb ratios, or correction factors.*

For one thing, if you rely on a given CGM reading to automatically trigger an appropriate insulin injection, you probably want the measurement to be very accurate as CE said. At this point, is it accurate enough? The CGM error rate that I have personally experienced makes me answer negatively as to continual automatic injections, but you might feel differently.

CE said he may well go to the current closed-loop system when he changes to a compatible insulin pump, despite the misgivings he expressed. I guess that's why he's a "cutting edge" diabetic, and I'm not! This is a highly individualized decision so talk over any device potentials with your doctor, other qualified medical personnel, and those who care about you.

At the time of this writing, nothing has passed the efficacy test as a single implanted automatic sensor/insulin injection unit (amounting to an artificial pancreas), the available pump systems simply being receptive and responsive to signals from a separate CGM. This currently means affixing two units to your body, each with its own maintenance and periodic replacement requirements. I, personally, am not willing to deal with all of that, especially since I'm not in trouble on the A1C side of things. Of course, if you already use both the pump and CGM like CE, going with a closed-loop system may not present the same issues for you. Here's a little summary statement from Medical News Today:

Omnipod is a tubeless continuous insulin infusion device that works similarly to an insulin pump. People can use this medical device to help automate their rapid-acting insulin therapy.

Individuals can also combine Omnipod technology with a continuous glucose monitor to create a hybrid closed loop system, which can mimic the function of a healthy pancreas. Research suggests that these systems can help improve diabetes management and quality of life.

Here's more from the same source on advantages and disadvantages:

Pros

- *may improve diabetes management and quality of life*
- *removes the need for regular injections with a syringe or insulin pen*
- *provides more freedom*
- *stores data and useful information that can optimize management*
- *easy to use and automates many steps for monitoring blood glucose*

Cons

- *can be expensive if not available on insurance*
- *may create reliance on the technology*
- *may cause skin irritation where the cannula pierces the skin*
- *may fall off*
- *may cause device fatigue*

So we all, with the help of qualified physicians, must make our own decisions about using the technology available. No one shoe necessarily fits all. Examples mentioned herein are just that—examples!

What about the cure? My skeptical self has gone so far as to convince me that it will probably not be happening in my lifetime or maybe not in anyone's lifetime who lives another ten to twenty years.

You see, for at least a half-century, I have heard and read about the cure being "imminent". That's my best excuse for skepticism, but there's more added by the potential effect on a very profit-oriented pharmaceutical industry as mentioned by CE. What would a cure do to that industry?

While there is enough reason for skepticism, CE's updated comment on cure developments stopped skeptical me dead in my mental tracks! What do you think? Hey, for all we know, developments may be even further down the road to a cure by the time you read this! So, should I repeat this book's oft-repeated disclaimer/admonition, or do you automatically think of <u>running it by your doctor</u> by now? (underlined just in case)

Maybe my skeptical self should provide something more positive, so here goes!

As passed on through oral history, the cure actually happened—a very long time ago. Supposedly, a sailor and fellow crew members were caught in a storm at sea. Their ship was damaged. They ended up lost without navigation and rudder. and just drifted aimlessly for six months. The diabetic, whose expected life span was short in those days, only consumed cabbage and water.

The ship was finally found, and the diabetic sailor no longer had diabetes! He lived happily to a ripe old age. I suppose a wise guy could say, "Oh, sure, he didn't have diabetes when found because he was actually found dead! It is all fiction, or he never had the real deal, type 1 diabetes." All I'm saying is get your affairs in order before trying cabbage and water. (I tried to be positive!)

I still think we are more likely to see an artificial pancreas before a cure, perhaps a lot more likely! The Mayo Clinic actually refers to the current closed loop systems in artificial pancreas terms as follows:

The Food and Drug Administration has approved two artificial pancreases for people with type 1 diabetes who are age 14 and older. This is also called a closed loop system. The device, which is implanted in the body, links

*a continuous glucose monitor to an insulin pump. The
monitor checks blood sugar levels every five minutes.
The device automatically delivers the correct amount of
insulin when the monitor shows that it's needed.*

As highly as I regard Mayo, I do not consider any current
closed loop system, that I know of, to be an "artificial pancreas".
Also, there is a lot more to consider than the simple statement
above. Mayo goes into all of that, but here is a great way to
put it, this time provided by the Juvenile Diabetes Research
Foundation (JDRF), United Kingdom division:

*If you have type 1 diabetes, you already use treatment
loop – you measure your blood glucose levels, work out
how much insulin you need, then take a dose of insulin.
For this, you need a blood glucose meter, your brain,
and an insulin pen.*

*If you're using a hybrid closed loop system, you use a
CGM instead of a blood glucose meter, an insulin pump
instead of a pen, and an algorithm instead of your brain.*

*The CGM tells the algorithm what your glucose levels
are and the algorithm tells the pump how much insulin to
deliver. It will pause the flow of insulin if your levels are
low or increase the flow if your levels are high.*

*However, you will still need to check the system is
working. You'll also need to count carbs and be aware of
how quickly carbohydrate will reach your bloodstream,
so that you can give the system correct bolusing data
before you eat....*

...Hybrid closed loop or artificial pancreas?

*You may have heard this technology referred to as either
artificial pancreas or hybrid closed loop, or both.*

The Cutting-Edge Type 1 Diabetic

It's called the artificial pancreas because the system tries to replicate what the insulin-producing beta cells in the pancreas do in someone without type 1. Some people aren't happy with this, because it makes it sound like the person using an artificial pancreas has the equivalent of a fully functioning pancreas, which isn't true because it still takes effort to make sure the system works properly.

Also, the pancreas does other things besides regulating glucose which aren't affected by having type 1 diabetes – so the pancreas is still doing part of its job.

Some people prefer to say hybrid closed loop; 'closed loop' because it closes the treatment loop as explained above, and 'hybrid' because you still need to manage some aspects manually, alongside the automated parts....

...The pros and cons of hybrid closed loop technology

The pros

Reducing the burden of type 1 diabetes decisions

By automating the treatment loop, hybrid closed loop systems can dramatically reduce the number of decisions you have to make every day.

With hybrid closed loop systems, you can spend more time with your glucose levels in range, with less effort. For example, if you have a hypo whilst sleeping, hybrid closed loop technology will temporarily turn off the delivery of insulin to minimise the time you spend below target range. Your insulin will also be slowed or turned off if the sensor detects that glucose levels are likely to dip into a hypo.

Similarly, if the sensor detects that your glucose level is

*likely to rise above target, it will temporarily increase
the basal rate or deliver small corrective boluses – or a
combination of both.*

The cons

*Using a hybrid closed loop system eases the burden of
type 1 but doesn't mean that type 1 treatment is completely
automated. For example, you still need to count carbs
and give the system bolusing information when you eat.*

*You will still need to keep an eye on your glucose levels
and take action if the system isn't working properly, for
instance if your insulin infusion site isn't working well.
As you only use rapid acting insulin with a hybrid closed
loop system, you can quickly develop ketones if your
glucose rises and stays high due to technical issues.*

At first, in considering all of the information about what I
prefer to call the hybrid closed-loop systems available today,
I did a lot of research. Increasingly complicated, this pursuit
became more frustrating than it was worth so I yielded to the
quoting approach you've patiently waded through here. I just
hope you gain something factually constructive, and maybe even
get something from me offering my perspective in a transparent
way.

As I said before, regardless of what it's called, I personally
do not want to wear two separate devices and have to maintain
and replace them in short time increments. Plus, it could make
my rule of thumb approach to glucose levels become something
less flexible. However, I am not closed to going with the closed
loop in the future. I will stay open.

Even should integration of the two functions into one unit
become effective, CE's caution sign about accuracy, control, and
implantation might be my stop sign. I am one dull edge guy who
has concern about any automatic system being implanted in my

body. Potential problems seem too far beyond my control. Such a unit better be something proven well enough to generate a lot of confidence. Even if so, I would pray for God's power to infuse that unit—more faith in him than in it and the science behind it! That's just me, but I again urge you to run your considerations about these systems by your doctor or diabetic health care professional. You are an individual and never a ditto of me or anyone else! For all I know, you may find that the system I avoid is the one you should embrace!

As for the ever elusive "cure", bring it on! I am ready, but I do understand that an old guy like me can't be prioritized or considered before the children or others. In fact, I have no problem yielding to anyone at all. If it is presented one day, to God be the glory just as I credit him for all I'm worth, even to the point of the cross.

How do you feel about all of this? I bet you are going to do something more edgy, or—at least—continue the discussion with your doctor and others, staying open. Here's a bit of advice about the cutting edge that I am not hesitant to share: Never say never! Last, but not least, one more thing applies for sure to this stuff. Sometimes, we feel so insignificant, but it's not true. God knows you and me, and he values us!

Are not two sparrows sold for a penny? Yet not one of them will fall to the ground outside your Father's care. And even the very hairs of your head are all numbered. So don't be afraid; you are worth morethan many sparrows (Matthew 10:29-31).

5

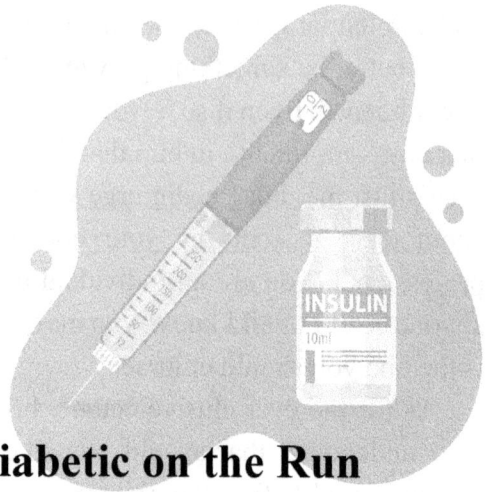

The Diabetic on the Run

Me and my CGM—

In this chapter, I will again be doing my best to use my own experience as an example—far from a perfect one but, hopefully, transparent and humanly imperfect in a way that provides good food for thought. Your experience may very well be different, and I'm guessing that your example isn't perfect either!

My planning on the run, variable adjustments, or audibles (football quarterback changing the play called) became more frequent with the CGM. If adjusting food, exercise, and insulin on the run more effectively meant wearing a CGM, I would gladly do it. Guess what happened? I did, and it worked! Previously, my average A1C readings were in the 7.5 to 8.2 range. After going with the CGM (Dexcom 5, 6 and now 7), the range became 6.4 to 6.8, over a full point lower with more consistency as well!

Of course, the CGM has no magical ability to transform glucose levels. That's where I and my lifestyle audibles come in. It's all about my willingness to adjust readily and how I adjust those all-important variables in response to CGM readings: 1. diet, 2. exercise, and ....3. insulin

Through my 50s, sports was a big variable, but not always well-timed or accurately amenable to glucose readings. Of course, those readings (finger sticks only—ouch!) were not available through a body attachment signaling my iPhone! In my 60s, the go-to exercise variable for me was running. In my 70s, it has become fast-walking in our hilly neighborhood. My routine (easier implementation in retirement) involves an early morning hilly walk of at least two miles, and weather permitting, a less consistent, more casual walk of maybe a mile in the early evening.

Regardless of routine, a high glucose reading certainly cannot simply prompt responsive, adequate exercise. Reading an out-of-whack number without responding on the run means absolutely zip! Drinking water has become more important to me, and begrudgingly cutting back on meal portions and/or content continues with high readings, but even in retirement, such variables are not always practical, given the circumstances.

Even given limitations on audible calls, note that making insulin dosage adjustments is a distant third on the variable list. That's because the first two are superior in terms of collateral benefits, and they are less risky than adjusting insulin dosage. They are my normal go-to adjustments unless there are extenuating circumstances, and—even then—adjustments of insulin on the run, for me, should be very conservative in order to avoid hyper and especially hypoglycemic risk.

In addition to others, one extenuating circumstance could be an extremely high glucose level that can't be reasonably modified by using either or both of the first two adjustments. Again, it is extremely important to remember that such things are highly individualized so discuss your adjustment plan thinking (or audible calling potentials) with your doctor or qualified medical professional.

In fact, before we go further into the mysterious and questionably sane area of my personal diabetic life, maybe I can find a creative way to repeat what I have said repeatedly: I am me, not you. You are you, and your you probably does not exactly fit my me in terms of struggling with diabetes. (We do ruminate about such brainy stuff!) Your life is indeed yours, and the only good reason that we venture into mine is to provide some constructive food for thought.

In my case, I take one long-acting insulin dose (Lantus) in the morning and one prior to my evening meal plus a fast-acting dose (Novolog) before each of three meals—a total of five injections a day. I used to take only one of the Lantus injections a day. That was before my doctor recommended splitting it into am and pm doses due to problems controlling high glucose levels in the morning, basically fasting levels. This is sometimes called the "dawn phenomenon". It is not phenomenal if that means really great. In this instance, it means that it's just puzzling!

We won't let the dawn phenomenon hang. There will be more, less puzzling content regarding it in a later chapter. Anyway, the split dosage adjustment plus a few more evening units helped a great deal. It's a good example of how we benefit by keeping our medical professionals informed. They sometimes may be able to help us struggle in very practical ways!

Some type 1 diabetics take fewer daily injections and some more per individual plans worked out with their doctors. However, I have discovered that the number of injections does not necessarily tell you anything about how much insulin is injected daily. It's a highly individualized matter.

While I take five injections, the total number of U-100 units I inject daily varies some due to fast-acting Novolog which I vary a few units prior to each meal depending on the CGM reading (mine on my iPhone) and the anticipated meal plus exercise. I have found that my variations may be more or less than another diabetic, regardless of the number of injections.

I do occasionally (maybe a few times a week) take an extra injection, but for me, a conservative rule of thumb makes it contingent on a very high glucose level with no foreseeable imminent exercise. When that occurs, I may take a low dose of fast-acting insulin, rarely over 5 units and generally 3-4 units. That's because a PA and I figured that 1 unit of Novolog fast-acting insulin usually results in about a 40 point lowering of my glucose level, all other factors remaining constant. (As always, my usual may be your unusual.)

With 40 points per unit in mind and no exercise or meal foreseen, a stable (with no up or down arrow per the CGM) glucose reading of 250 would not prompt administration of 5 units because that could, in turn, prompt a glucose outcome of 50 (250 minus 200 or 5x40). That's hypoglycemia and way too low to go! The low glucose alarm on my CGM would be going crazy, and I would be experiencing those disgusting hypo symptoms!

The way I would go is to take no more than 3 units when the glucose reading is 250, usually resulting in an outcome of about 130, well above hypoglycemic danger. (250 minus 120 or 3x40). That allows some room for an unpredictable variance. If a pre-bedtime night glucose reading is below 250, I put up with it unless and until awakened by my CGM excessive glucose warning, a number I can set myself per a chosen maximum. With the Lantus evening adjustment mentioned before, my normal sleeping glucose will be going down slowly, but that is not set in stone by any means.

Most folks don't need help in determining what to do when glucose gets too far down (consume glucose tablets, juice, sugared soft drinks, candy, other high-sugar products). However, I have learned that our individualism includes differing physical sensitivity to low glucose signals. If I don't pick it up physically, my CGM will, and it will alert or alarm me in response to pre-set scores—just as it will for my chosen high limits. My Dexcom 6 CGM had a mandatory low alarm that I could only avoid by shutting off my phone. The Dexcom 7 has other delaying options, but the default (in effect, emergency) setting of 55 is the same.

One thing I have learned about using the continuous glucose monitor is that the advice coming with the monitor is solid, i.e.

"watch and wait". If I have some doubt about the accuracy of a high reading and it's not ridiculously high (for me, 275 or up), I will do just that to see if the trending continues upward. However, after so long, I am pretty familiar with high glucose feelings so, if my feelings are aligned with the number, my trust level may be good enough to act on it—always with insulin as the last alternative move.

I do not wait and watch much when it comes to low readings, not trusting my feelings as much due to the relative danger. Of course, it may prompt consumption of something like a glucose-raising food, drink, or snack (Glucagon injection if necessary). In my case, if what I just consumed is not kicking in yet, I may well wait and watch the number to verify the expected upward trend. New readings appear every five minutes on my CGM.

As an undergraduate in college, my most memorable low glucose response was one that illustrates a couple of things discussed previously. At the time, my roommate and I lived in a rented garage apartment, complete with its own kitchen. I had a meal contract elsewhere, but he enjoyed cooking his meals at the apartment.

One day, during a break in classes, I was alone at the apartment when an extreme hypoglycemic episode hit me faster than usual. For some unremembered reason, I did not have a sugar remedy nearby so naturally I opened the refrigerator. There, in all its glory, was a freshly made lemon icebox pie, all of which I rapidly consumed. Passing out was no option!

My roommate arrived immediately after my over-consumption episode, finding me still in a groggy state and unable to communicate clearly. He called 911, and an ambulance arrived shortly. They insisted that it was necessary to transfer me to the emergency room, though I was already feeling much better. On the trip, I was lucid and feeling great—great enough to insist that I was fine, even joking with the EMTs. Type 1 diabetics know how quickly we recover.

The Diabetic on the Run

After returning home that night, I did not feel lousy, but it was only because the ER Physician used insulin to counteract the extreme influx of sugar into my body via an entire pie! Otherwise, I would have been miserable since the effects of extreme glucose swings, low-to-high in this case, will do that. By the way, to this day, my friend holds the lemon-pie incident jokingly over my head. I guess good friends (of mine at least) know they need to use whatever they've got to keep good friends in line!

Let's just say that it was, and is, so easy to go too far in response. We can feel so hungry, but we are usually not on the brink of starvation, though we may feel like it! In this case, one slice would have sufficed! That was in the 1960s. Today, we don't have an easy excuse for such overcompensation in that CGMs give us a much-needed look at the running effect on our glucose levels.

One of the Dexcom features already mentioned has been very helpful along these lines. Beginning with the G6 and continuing with the G7, it's a trending arrow beside the glucose number (pointing up, down, or in a neutral direction). For me, it is generally trustworthy, apart from some reservations as mentioned before. The G7 is a smaller, single injectable mechanism containing both sensor and transmitter (separate installation with G6) and much less time from attachment to activation (30 minutes compared to G6's 2 hours).

The Dexcom model's accuracy continues to improve as it did from the G5 to G6 models. No matter the claim in that regard, I still do periodic calibrations by finger stick. Of course, there are other CGM systems, and some things vary from brand to brand. However, a lot of the principles and practicalities are the same. I can only testify to the fact that the CGM systems I have used have certainly helped me maintain much better control— struggling better, one aspect being a big improvement in calling those quarterback audibles each day at the line of scrimmage. I rarely yell those out, you know!

Maybe I will be an all-star quarterback—in my dreams! It's the long run that counts, and focusing on the right thing is key. One thing for sure helps me see progress or set-backs day-to-day, as intended:

Therefore do not worry about tomorrow, for tomorrow will worry about itself. Each day has enough trouble of its own. But seek first his kingdom and his righteousness, and all these things will be given to you as well (Matthew 6:33-34).

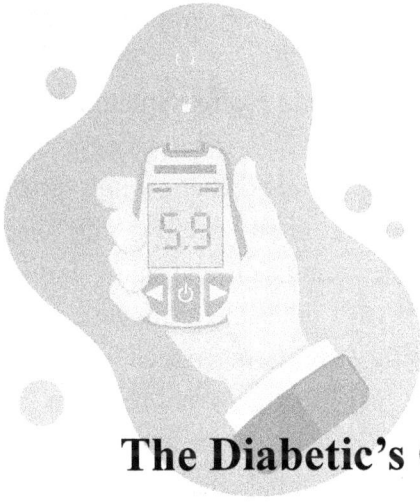

6

The Diabetic's Good Doctor

Remember cutting edge CE? I gave him a bonus question about doctors:

If you assembled a reasonable list of questions to pose to a diabetic specialist as your prospective doctor, what would they be?

(For type 2 folks: When considering what CE says and a lot of other things to follow, try substituting type 2 for type 1.)

CE: *Disclaimer: I currently see my primary care doctor for my diabetes management for convenience and cost reduction. However, for much of my diabetes journey I saw an endocrinologist.*

A. Do you have other patients for whom you help manage Type 1 diabetes?
B. Do you have Type 1 diabetes or personally know someone (friend or family member) with Type 1 diabetes?
C. Do you have other patients who use insulin pumps and/ or CGMs?
D. What is your philosophy on how to best manage Type 1 diabetes?
E. How often would you want to see me for regular diabetes

checkups, assuming my A1C and other lifestyle aspects are in decent control?

CE's disclaimer is pretty good. Convenience and cost reduction are important factors we weigh in choosing a doctor, but don't forget that CE is a cutting-edge diabetic whose glucose is well controlled, and he isn't necessarily dealing with exactly the same issues you or I may be facing. A friend said I should be seeing an Endocrinologist. It isn't unusual for diabetics to use an Internist or maybe a Family Practitioner rather than a more specialized Endocrinologist. My doctor is an Internist right now, but I certainly have nothing against those more specialized physicians. I had one once. For some diabetics, they may be the best doctors but not for me right now.

When I considered the insulin pump, my Internist at the time referred me to an Endocrinologist. He felt it best because the specific concerns I had exceeded his expertise, and I appreciated that. When I decided against the pump for reasons very specific to me and my unique life circumstances, I just continued to see my Internist. I call that good medical practice and decent consumerism on my part, too. Currently, I have the doctor who helps me best considering my current needs, financial realities, location, etc.

My experience is that a lot of my former doctors knew a lot about diabetes, but some did not tell me what I need to know, that is, according to my individual needs and unique circumstances. However, I cannot blame the doctors. I think my reason for not assigning a bunch of blame is pretty sound: It's me! Here's what I mean:

First, let's agree that we should think of doctors as God-given blessings, but they are human, imperfect like you and me. Now, how should we view ourselves as patients? You see, for a long time, I did not view myself as a consumer who considered healthcare as a vital product for which I paid dearly. I was more like one of many subjects over whom doctors reigned! He or she knew all, and I knew nothing. The doctor spoke. I listened. I practically genuflected before them! This was no doctor's fault.

There were few, if any, questions coming from my end of the deal, and doctors rarely knew much at all about my day-to-day existence on God's good earth. While we have a lot in common, you understand that your daily life is not the same as mine. A doctor only knows what we are willing to reveal about ourselves. Remember the chapter on transparency?

I would say that the most positive turn in being able to truly take advantage of what doctors had to offer this diabetic was actually two turns. The first was becoming a consumer. The second was becoming a transparent consumer. The first was much easier, for me, than the second!

Once, on moving to a new city, I found a qualified doctor who, due to what I shared with him, found a great playing field on which to challenge and coach me up. It was my avid interest in sports and sports competition. He was also a sports nut, and proposed that we approach my diabetes struggle as a competition.

My opponent was me, and the doctor was my coach. If nothing else, we had a common language to use with each other, an enthusiastic one, and he did not hesitate to use it! We talked about football almost as much as we did about the Big D! It may not seem therapeutic, but it was just that. My competitive nature got in gear as we talked glucose levels and quarterback audibles, even though, at that time, glucose scores were determined only with point-in-time blood test strips and those irritating finger pricks!

We lived in that location for a few years, and I only had four appointments with this good doctor. However, he helped me big time in the long run. I learned that a good doctor's treatment plan was as much a product of knowing me as it was knowing the subject of diabetes or any other serious condition I carried around. Still, it must be recognized as much easier said than done for most doctors today.

Living with Diabetes

Now, please understand that the football deal was very unusual—a rare find. Beyond those appointments, doctors using terms like "audible" and "touchdown" were nonexistent. I do not expect anything even remotely like that from a doctor. I'm not saying one or two didn't say something like Roll Tide! (Sorry, but seven years attending an institution, a lot of games, and countless shouts of support for many years reinforce such stuff in me.)

My point with all of this is that a good doctor helped me know that my individualism could factor into my treatment. Information about me as a person mattered. For the purposes of this chapter, I reviewed a list of my doctors over the years. After leaving home for college, I lived in 5 different cities in 3 states, and had a total of 8 primary physicians, 4 of those after football guy. I can't say that any of them have been as much fun, but I can say that I have not encountered one that wasn't good, one caveat considered—my input as a transparent consumer!

I have five of my own suggestions to share along the lines of good doctors for diabetics, all or some of which you may be able to use:

1. Pray for the doctor you need.
2. If possible, find a doctor, nurse, PA, or even a diabetes educator who can be very down to earth and willing to talk about all aspects of this lifestyle physical and mental struggle. Not that we should find a doctor or health professional who leads us down the lifestyle path—just someone bringing their expertise and work on our behalf down the trail we blaze. We are the transparent consumers! Beyond my football doctor appointments, some of the most productive appointments were with a Physician's Assistant (PA). He was a type 1 diabetic like me (big bonus as CE said), and was practical in sharing his experience and relating it to mine. Together, we came to some important conclusions.

3. <u>If possible, network to find the best doctor and/or health professional for you</u>! For my current doctor, I used Facebook Messenger for local friends, and Nextdoor.com for my area where I found references already provided due to a previous posted request for doctors treating diabetics. I also checked out different rating services and patient reviews online—not just one site. Of course, I also sought input from a few non-Facebook friends. An initial list of five doctors was narrowed to a short list of three due to location convenience. Of course, everybody's own factors affect narrowing.

4. <u>Ask questions up front, and establish your intent to be a transparent consumer</u>! Don't worry about setting yourself up for failure. Your doctor will likely know that you are an imperfect human, don't you think? Fortunately, the first one I visited after the narrowing process has always seemed well suited, answered my questions well, and was receptive to my transparent consumer proposition.

5. <u>If possible, find a professional who is willing to meet you on your own unique playing field as laid out by you! Again, I know they are busy so be proactive</u>! You could prepare for the first appointment by thinking things through and even writing down or dictating thoughts about yourself and diabetes (including habits and medications) on your phone. Whether you give it to your professional or just discuss it with him or her is up to you, but transparency is key!

Maybe my post-diabetes first doctor story will help in thinking about the playing field and doctors. It's for all, but if you or someone you love is a young diabetic, I ask you to especially listen up.

I was diagnosed with diabetes by a small-town GP at age twelve, and resided for two long weeks in a hospital at The University of Alabama, Birmingham or UAB—an excellent facility. The idea was to synchronize treatment and attitudes to an insulin regimen and my new life reality. I was formally diagnosed with diabetes mellitus—not called type 1 then—remember, no 2, no 1!

My specialist at UAB hospital was a doctor whose name was such that it could be cruelly amusing when pronounced in a corrupted way. It did not take me long to begin using the corrupted version. He was just so serious, and the most memorable look on his face could be imitated by sucking on a lemon. He was smart and himself a diabetic—type 1. Needless to say, he had a lot to offer.

I did not like him from the get-go, especially since I bordered on depression and cried myself to sleep some nights during the two weeks I was in the hospital. After all, I was twelve years old and from a small town a million miles away or so it felt. I honestly thought this doctor should have been a Funeral Director (sorry for stereotyping Funeral Directors, but I repeat my best excuse—age 12!).

I know—I was bad—but look, comedic relief had helped me block out a lot of family struggles, and I had to get my jollies any way I could! As a diabetic himself, the doc was uniquely positioned to use his experience as part of an effective bedside manner, and a little levity can be downright therapeutic—no comedian needed, just an occasional smile and a tad of humor. Of course, some of my disdain for this doctor probably came from projection. As a counselor years later, I saw plenty of that! I'm sure the doctor did his best and cared. He just needed a little work on showing it and individualizing his bedside manner.

Oh, I know that the "experts" are not necessarily going to be able to meet you on that unique practical ground where you are based—your home field. Your home field is your uniqueness—your psyche, your body, your spirit, your life, even your style. They don't have time. They can't know everybody. Yes, but I do believe they should try. A halfway alert patient knows when a doctor is not trying.

The Diabetic's Good Doctor

The funny name doctor was indeed an "expert" and himself diabetic, but how close could he get to walking in my shoes? That is a crucial question because, when it comes to such things as attitudes and those ever-elusive variables I mentioned before, a good doctor must see you as the unique individual God created. In my view, a good doctor or other qualified medical professional is someone who puts some effort into searching for you—as an individual—not someone assuming a lot. You and I just need to do our parts to help them see us.

As I said, some nights in that hospital, I cried myself to sleep. It was not so much crying about the Big D as about being far from home with nobody to hang with me while I struggled. In the hospital, nurses came in periodically during the night to make sure I had not dropped off the deep end when it came to the ever-precarious balance between glucose and insulin. They would even wake me up to get readings. At least once, a nurse came in when I was crying. I quickly buried my head in my pillow, and stifled the sobs. I never told anyone how miserable I felt during those long nights—well into my adulthood. In my family, feelings were generally not a topic of discussion.

One consolation was that a few of those nurses were bombshells—beautiful with smiles to match and caring too! At age twelve, I was—so to speak—starting to feel my oats. I had never had a date, and had no idea which way was up or down in terms of male-female relationships. However, I knew and appreciated a beautiful woman when I saw one! In fact, the more I thought about it later, the more I realized that this was one of the more therapeutic aspects of my time in that hospital. Nurses can sometimes indeed compensate for doctors' shortcomings— sour lemons, lack of individualizing, whatever. Thank God for good nurses and PAs!

Okay, so they are individuals like us, and a doctor without a bedside sense of humor might suit some of us just fine. I just want him or her to have a little bit of humor to offer people like me, even more so with bewildered kids! In my adult case, I want to see a doctor at least occasionally chuckle with me and listen very well—to the point of showing some ability to reword my concerns right back at me.

A doctor does not have to see things exactly as I do, but he or she should be able to yield to me on some things, especially since—in my case—I may just know a thing or two about their science and how it relates to my uniqueness. I want to know if a doctor is so clinical as to bypass common sense. A doctor who considers his or her treatment of diabetes to be an exact science is not realistic enough for me. For instance, I once had a doctor who told me that I could maintain a consistent graph level of glucose scores that varied only slightly—ha! Fortunately, he later learned better.

My current doctor is no jokester, but he is an excellent listener and manages to chuckle at some of my quirky stuff occasionally. He once mentioned that my blood pressure was a bit elevated. It had been taken by the nurse just before he arrived. I said I thought it must be white coat syndrome since that had proven to be the case before. As he was leaving the room, he said he would have the nurse come in to check my blood pressure again. I said, "Now that I told you about white coat syndrome, you would tell me she's coming in!" He chuckled and said, "Well, she might or might not come in." I laughed, appreciated the humor, and—no—I don't expect it every visit.

Advice: Your life is not permanently soured. You can have type 1 or type 2 and live a good, sweet life for a long time so loosen up and appreciate it when your doctor loosens up! I also try to consider that the one rendering a service to me probably benefits from my consideration and even some of my humor at any given time, and things like asking about their day is part of my role as a good patient.

I don't want to be overly repetitious, but sometimes, we might find it challenging to apply the charge quoted below to our relationships with certain people. Some doctors might be among them. This is certainly something Jesus said that deserves repeating a lot anyway:

Do to others as you would have them do to you (Luke 6:31).

We should be considerate, but we should also continue to ask questions about our treatment, including any recommendations, especially justification for medications and dosage adjustments. If they can't explain why it is the correct path, maybe we should go back to the short list. If they are unwilling to discuss lifestyle, diet, exercise, all aspects of individual health, and instead they simply want to medicate us, we should definitely move on—again, with that huge caveat: Before working ourselves into a consumer lather, let's make sure we expect as much of ourselves by initiating discussions about this stuff as transparent consumers. In my experience, the good doctor wants to hear it and wants to be responsive—funny thing though: Every doctor I have ever known has been 100% human!

Exercise common sense at all times, and please do not settle for less than good care. Consequences for mis-treatment or missed treatment are severe. You will find a doctor who is worthy of treating you as you do your part. They are out there. We sure need them. It's neat that God even inspired a physician to record what Jesus had to say about how the medical and spiritual aspects of our need relate!

Jesus answered them, "It is not the healthy who need a doctor, but the sick" (Luke 5:31).

7

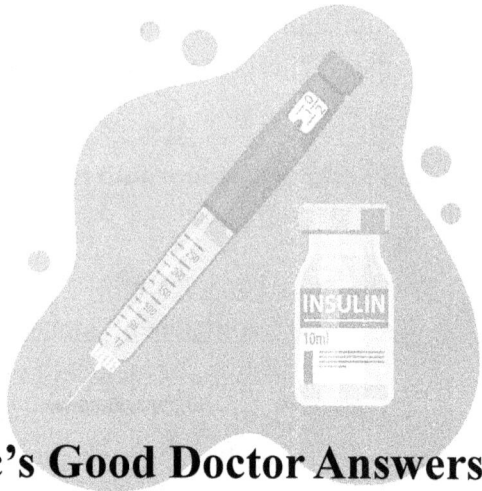

The Diabetic's Good Doctor Answers Important Questions

Some good information will be found in the answers received to probing questions submitted to an experienced Internist whom I will call MD. This doctor prefers to remain anonymous. The option was offered due to the high level of transparency requested. This physician has a lot of experience with demographically diverse populations and with diabetics, both types. The responses here are concise and to the point. (When not specified, questions apply to both type 1 and type 2 diabetes.)

1. What has prepared you to treat diabetes successfully?

MD - *I stay current with diabetes management through regular medical journal updates and online reading/continuing medical education.*

2. What are the greatest challenges you have faced in attempting to treat type 1 diabetes successfully? What about type 2?

MD - *Greatest challenge by far is dealing with medication costs.*

3. In treating diabetes (type 1 and/or 2), what are the primary medical system or insurance factors that may affect the prospect of successful treatment?

MD - *Coverage of medications and cost.*

4. In your experience, do diabetics sometimes manifest forms of denial that limit successful self-regulation?

MD - *There are always people who don't want to recognize their diagnosis of diabetes type 2. This obviously doesn't really happen with type 1 diabetics. Many type 2 diabetics don't have symptoms so they may not accept that something is wrong.*

5. Please suggest a list of questions that a patient could apply to any given doctor in order to determine if that doctor will be able to help him or her manage diabetes successfully.

MD - *Do you stay current with diabetes management recommendations? Will your staff help with prior authorizations for medications? What diabetic resources are available through your clinic?*

6. In a perfect treatment world, what would be different in your treatment of diabetes?

MD - *I could prescribe any appropriate medication and insurance would cover it. I could have staff that could call poorly controlled diabetics every few weeks to review glucoses and discuss plans.*

7. In a perfect response world, what would be different in your diabetic patients' response?

MD - *Basically agree to recommended medication regimens and comply with diet/exercise recommendations*

8. In your opinion, why did type 2 become a medical diagnosis?

MD - *A population that has increasingly become more obese.*

9. What is your opinion regarding the efficacy of CGM systems available today?

MD - *CGM's are a game changer. They should be available to every diabetic.*

10. In your opinion, why is there not yet a cure for type 1? Do you think such a cure is imminent?

MD - *I think a cure would be extremely difficult as you'd need to find a way to make genetic changes to an individual. I don't see something like that available in the next century.*

I find words inadequate to express how much I appreciate this good doctor answering these important questions. Again, your analysis of the answers is probably as good as mine, but you can't comment here so I'm providing some comment food for your brain below—you know, food for thought? Of course, the garbage bin option is still available!

In regard to preparation for treating diabetes successfully, I would add experience specific to diabetes to the list because this doctor has certainly had a lot of it. MD apparently interpreted the denial question as more of an absolute, i.e. "Fredish"-like form, rather than the subtle forms discussed earlier—as practiced by "part-time" deniers like me! I had not considered how pervasive the more absolute form may be among type 2 diabetics, especially those without symptoms. It makes sense. Assuming that none of us are absolute deniers, we need to keep our helping antennae out for those folks and gently help them face their diagnoses.

I especially like the idea of asking doctors about "diabetic resources" available. Also, what a great thing it would be for staff to stay in touch with patients whose diabetic regulation is especially challenging. That might seem to be a pipe dream. However, participating in a group or comparing notes with other diabetics is not. It is another viable way to get support and feedback while giving the same! As for cure prospects, this good doctor is even more of a skeptic than me!

The good doctor's repeated answers as to lack of adequate insurance or other financial coverage reinforced something in my consideration—being considerate of those without needed resources. In fact, I must say that I stood convicted as soon as I read these responses. I am able to access the resources needed to successfully regulate my diabetes, but some diabetics may not be so fortunate. I have not given the needs of those people enough attention. The doctor is spot-on, and a big part of the self-regulating resources needed, but not available for many, is the "game changer" continuous glucose monitor (CGM) that "should be available to every diabetic". It has certainly proven to be a key for me.

There have been recent initiatives in making this game changing CGM affordable for more people in the United States by expanding Medicare and Medicaid coverage eligibility. Check out the following excerpt from an article published by the American Diabetes Association (ADA):

March 2, 2023: Centers for Medicare and Medicaid Services (CMS) Announce Expanded Continuous Glucose Monitor (CGM) Coverage.

CMS announced expanded coverage of continuous glucose monitors (CGMs) to include all insulin-dependent people and those with a history of problematic hypoglycemia.

"The American Diabetes Association (ADA) has been a leader in advocating for broader access to important

diabetes technology for all people living with diabetes. We applaud CMS' decision allowing for all insulin-dependent people as well as others who have a history of problematic hypoglycemia to have access to a continuous glucose monitor, a potentially life-saving tool for diabetes management," said Chuck Henderson, Chief Executive Officer, American Diabetes Association. "Making this resource more widely available is a critical objective of the ADA's Technology Access Project, and we will continue to press for policies that ensure all people with diabetes, especially those who are under-resourced, have access to life-saving technologies."...

This is not to say that we should leave such a matter in the hands of our government. It's just my opinion, but I think I'm among many Christians who believe that we may have too often allowed government to be a substitute for our God-given responsibilities toward others. There is much more to do in this regard and in other areas of resource availability for diabetics. Christians like me need to understand this and help others with it as opportunities appear, regardless of status.

Given my background, I should never ignore the needs of other diabetics less fortunate than me. Given my salvation, there is no absolutely no excuse. I may have been oblivious to their needs, but I'm always able to determine to change, ask for forgiveness, and make that change with God's help. My change begins right here on this page. God loves us and those around us!

For I was hungry and you gave me nothing to eat, I was thirsty and you gave me nothing to drink, I was a stranger and you did not invite me in, I needed clothes and you did not clothe me, I was sick and in prison and you did not look after me.' "They also will answer, 'Lord, when did we see you hungry or thirsty or a stranger or needing clothes or sick or in prison,

and did not help you?' "He will reply, 'Truly I tell you, whatever you did not do for one of the least of these, you did not do for me' (Matthew 25:42-45).

8

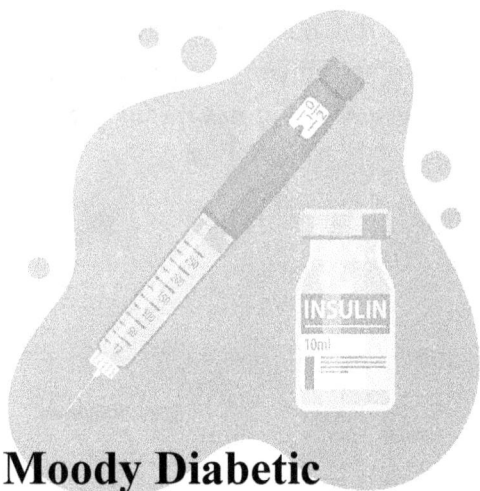

The Moody Diabetic

Another reason for my initial diabetes specialist's lack of humor could be the fact that he was a diabetic—no kidding! Here comes another one of those important quotes from a pretty good source (healthline.com), and it involves important things doctors may not often discuss:

> *...You may think Diabetes just affects your pancreas, but living with this condition often affects your mood and mental health too. For one, you may experience mood swings when your blood glucose levels are too high or low. Stress, depression, and anxiety can also crop up....*

Doctors can't pinpoint some of these things very readily when they reach a critical mass, so to speak, especially if we don't tell them about it. Still, I wish someone had given me a clue about this when I first got diabetes. I was 12, and pretty muted with doctors—parents too! For many years, no one did or—if someone did—it was not given enough emphasis to make an impression. That includes some pretty good doctors! Early on, maybe a lot was assumed since I had an older brother (away from home by the time I was a kid) with the big D. At any rate, I learned about the emotional/mood effects of diabetes the hard way.

The Moody Diabetic

Personally, my current experience of low and high effects starts at about 75 for a low and 200 for a high. At the low end, I definitely begin to experience weakness and get very quiet. At the high end, I'm out of sorts and negative, but usually put on a decent show. A good show is a no-show at the low end! I don't mess around with lows. We will take a closer look at low and high physical effects later.

There is some pretty practical advice from another resource, *New Life Outlook - Diabetes*. I advise that you <u>follow the advice quoted below</u>: (For some reason, I find the hands up metaphor at the end hilarious!)

....The following are our top six suggestions to keep mood swings at bay:

1. Work hard at a balanced carb diet. This will differ for each individual so be sure to talk to your doctor or dietician to understand what they are expecting from you.

2. Keep an emergency pack with you at all times in case of low blood sugar. This can come in the form of a granola bar, hard candy or glucose tablets. I keep some in my car and in my purse just in case I get stuck in traffic or at an appointment and can feel myself crashing.

3. Get off the couch. Seriously, if you have diabetes, it's IMPERATIVE to incorporate some type of exercise into your day. Start slowly if you have to — even just walking in place in front of the TV will make a difference. If you're tech-savvy, get a Fitbit or other step tracker. It's fun to challenge your friends (and yourself) and see what you can do.

4. Yoga, meditation and mindfulness are really helpful at calming your emotions. There are many free meditation videos available on YouTube.

5. Track your sugar levels. If you are catching yourself in a mood and you know it, take the time to take a reading. If you can get a handle on whether you are going too low or too high in your counts, it will give you a better idea of how to solve the problem.

6. Talk to your doctor. If you are finding mood swings and feelings of depression/anxiety taking over your day, it might be time to get professional intercession. Your doctor can help you determine if your diet might be to blame, or if you need some depression medications, and they may even point you to a counselor to help you sort out your feelings.

Yes, diabetes is a burden and not an easy one to bear. But with education, careful planning, and some creative solutions, you can tackle the emotional roller coaster and ride with your hands up.

I learned a lot about diabetes-related emotional stuff in my twenties, but probably was in my forties before I admitted to myself its true effects on me. Even today, I sometimes underestimate it. Facing it early would have helped since the psyche is subject to habit formation, and old habits in thinking are harder to break than relatively young thinking habits. My advice on this is <u>own the mood effects a.s.a.p. and communicate it to those who provide you with medical care, but especially family and those who care about you.</u>

Even in my forties, I rarely ever talked about my feelings. Talking about my diabetes was even less likely. I was too "macho" to own up to emotions or mood swings I couldn't control. For me, a lot of that was wrapped up in effects from my early family and culture life. Believe me, the men around me did not talk emotions at all. As a boy, I caught on to that fast. To talk about emotions was tantamount to being a "sissy"!

The Moody Diabetic

I have found, from years of stifling followed by opening up more, that there is a lot of power in literally calling this stuff out. Yes, if we own it for ourselves and with others, the best interests of both will usually be best served! They want to understand, and it will help them be patient. You will find it easier to be patient with yourself too.

I can honestly say that my progress in dealing with the emotional end of the Big D is amazing over the last few decades. It is worth repeating: I have found that seeing my diabetes for what it is and calling it out before myself, others, and God - actually verbally, out-loud (not too loud you understand) is key. "I'm feeling pretty negative right now. The old glucose is up." Facing it and sharing it is important to reasonably controlling it—not perfect control but reasonable control. For type 1, that elusive break through to an average A1C level of below 7 is doable or to whatever level is a realistic and ambitious goal for anyone—either type!

I am not generally depressed as a result of high glucose levels, but I usually feel less positivity and more socially inhibited. Sometimes, not due so much to feelings, but more due to long-term high glucose effects, I need to drink lots of water and go for a walk if possible, and if it escalates too much, try to diminish my glucose level by a conservative (usually a few units) dose of fast acting insulin. It bears repeating that one reason for a conservative extra insulin approach is not to go from one extreme to another. The worst of bad diabetic days for me have been when that has happened—high to low or low to high in a short time.

Of course, apart from mood swings generated by varying glucose levels, there's the emotional effects of the struggle itself. You don't have to be a former mental health professional like me to know that mental health is a highly individual thing. Just as every diabetic struggles with diabetes, every human being struggles with something, usually more than one something. It's called life!

Sometimes, we just reach boiling points. The following information and good advice comes from the American Diabetes

Association. You can substitute any number of other physical struggles and adjustments for the term *diabetes* and its adjustments portrayed here—right? (Note the emphasis on openness/transparency.)

With diabetes, you have a lot on your mind.

Tracking your blood sugar levels, dosing insulin, planning your meals, staying active—it's a lot to think about. It can leave you feeling run down, emotionally drained and completely overwhelmed. It's called diabetes burnout. And that's why it's important to stay in touch with your emotions as you manage your diabetes. What are you feeling? Stressed out? Angry? Sad? Scared? Take time to take inventory of your emotions and reach out to those around you to talk honestly and openly about how you feel.

Better yet, find a mental health care provider to guide you through the emotional terrain around your disease and discover ways to lighten your mental load. With diabetes, feeling physically good is half the battle. Feeling mentally good is the other half.

One big lesson I have learned is that I need to get as much humor from diabetes as I can without losing my focus on struggling effectively. One of the best tools in my bag is the ability to find humor and appreciate it—laugh about it.

I especially enjoy seeing the funny things about me and my struggle. It really does not take a lot of effort. If you are humorless about it, I don't see the future in me trying to get you to find a sense of humor. Either you have it or you don't, but if you can laugh at much of anything in your life, what do you have to lose from laughing at diabetes—actually at yourself as a diabetic?

Laughter is one of the best figurative medications I take. It helps me counter negativity and even mood effects from glucose extremes or just the daily grind of managing diabetes.

Blessed are you who hunger now, for you will be satisfied. Blessed are you who weep now, for you will laugh (Luke 6:21).

9

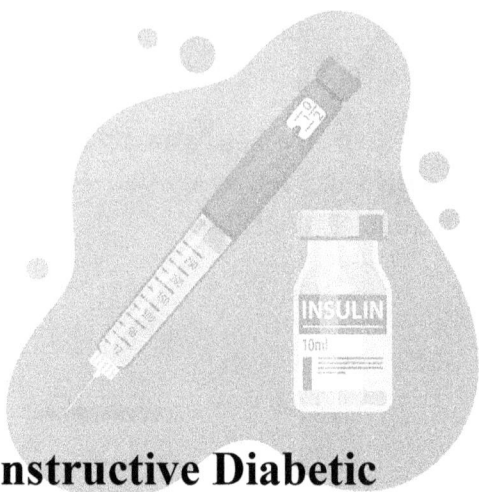

The Constructive Diabetic

One thing I know for sure: No matter how challenging it is to us as individuals, we all have concentration or focus choices. This chapter focuses on our focus!

During my inaugural hospitalization for diabetes at age 12, there was a girl in the hospital on another wing but not so far away. She was older than me—I think 15. She came in her wheelchair to visit me one of the first days I was there. It was a set up—had to be the work of those meddling nurses! I was alone and dumb enough to think I could hide being lonely, but those nurses knew. I thought they might have known when one of them came in the room, and I crammed my eyes full of tears into the pillow. She gently patted my back. The only reason I could not face the fact that the gig was up was that I was so good at hiding things from myself as I said before.

I can't remember exactly how this beautiful girl (even prettier than the prettiest nurse) explained why she came to visit me—something like she had heard I had checked in, and she wanted someone close to her age to talk to. I didn't care that it's a long way from 12 to 15, especially between a boy and girl (Yes, I buy the idea that girls mature sooner.)

She asked if I liked to play cards. My mom was an expert at all kinds of card games, and I had played a bunch with her so I was more than happy to accommodate. Over several days, we played a lot of card games in my room and in hers. I had a crush on her. She was a big reason I struggled well with downturns in mood.

Anyway, this neat story about the girl did not end well. One of my last days in the hospital, the nurse told me the girl was in bad shape. I knew she wasn't doing well a few days before when I visited her room. Her parents were there, and she had to stay in bed—no card games. I don't know if anyone ever told me what was wrong with her just as I don't remember her name. I was way too good at blocking things out and not opening up to talk about them. Would you believe I actually told that girl I cried one night? I remember that! She just had a way of getting things out of me—a friend I guess.

When the nurse told me this girl I had gotten to know was dying, I dropped right into my denial mode. She couldn't be that bad off. Just a few days ago, she beat me in double solitaire! I refused to let myself believe what the nurse was telling me. Then, she said that the girl would like to see me. I told her I really didn't feel like doing that right now. The next day, the girl died. I did not cry.

I came to know the truth. She came to see me in the first place because I was sad, and those scheming nurses thought it would be good for both of us to get to know each other—good for me because I needed a friend and good for her because she needed to be a friend to me. If that does not make sense to you, please think about this: We all need to find ways to quit staring at our own navels and see other people around us who want to be friends. In fact, we need to find those who need us to be their friends. Speaking of fact, this is sometimes a hard one: It is not all about me or you! (Okay, maybe this is a little preachy.)

If I had known Jesus Christ back then, I might have seen her, really seen her—in truth—in her good heart, and I think I would be more likely to remember that beautiful girl's name today. I like to think I would have had the heart to visit her. As a pretty immature twelve-year-old, I did not have what it takes to realize that it was not all about me.

To be honest, it took way too long for me to come to that realization. If you got it early, good for you! Now, I clearly see that not only is my diabetes not all about me, but also it has been important in the process that has made me who I am today. As imperfect as I am, I like being me! Here's some ways diabetes has helped make me a better person—far from perfect, but much better. I doubt anyone reading this would not want to grow in all of these areas.

*Purpose - As a Christian, I believe everything that happens in my life is a tool of God to mold me into the person he wants me to be. Even bad things are those tools. When I was diagnosed with the Big D at age 12, I did not believe this. Frankly, I did not have spiritual faith at all. If I had, I think it would have been an easier building process for me in terms of being equipped for the struggle.

Anyway, I am super glad that, by faith, I now see and appreciate God's purpose in anything and everything, whether I understand it or not—whether I like it or not. I don't like diabetes, but I do like some of the things I believe God has done and continues to do for me by using it.

While yours truly is far from being a star like type 1 diabetic and singer/actor Nick Jonas, I'm doing the same thing he did! He kept his diabetes on the QT before revealing it publicly for the good of others. He continues to do that as did Mary Tyler Moore (now deceased). Professional football quarterback Jay Cutler has done the same thing. How about type 2 folks? How about actress Halle Berry, actor Tom Hanks, and tennis pro Arthur Ashe (now deceased)? When these stars and others decided to open up about their diabetes to help others, a lot of us benefitted and still do. Writing this book is only part of that story for little old me!

The Constructive Diabetic

I consider myself blessed to use something personal like the big D to help others whenever the opportunity presents itself, mostly on a one-to-one basis. Hey, we don't have to be stars of any type to make a difference. We don't even have to be all-star diabetics—just fellow strugglers helping each other by sharing our struggles. Even openly admitting weaknesses can be helpful, not only to ourselves but also to fellow strugglers. We all want to know that we are not alone. A diabetic has great opportunity to serve others and glorify God!

But you are a chosen people, a royal priesthood, a holy nation, God's special possession, that you may declare the praises of him who called you out of darkness into his wonderful light (1 Peter 2:9).

*Discipline - Diabetes has helped me become a much more disciplined person than I ever would have been without it. My mother may have given me injections for a few years, but, entering my teen years not long after being diagnosed, I started feeling that I had been a mama's boy too long. That transition could have been delayed even further but for that diagnosis.

Like most adolescents, I actually wanted more independence, but being independent as a diabetic and just keeping my head above water called for more self-discipline than my life had provided me. Diabetes did not completely close that gap, but it definitely narrowed it. Self-discipline growth in my life got a big boost when I became a Christian. It was just in time since I was not far from tackling the challenge of parenthood. I needed help, and I got it!

For the Spirit God gave us does not make us timid, but gives us power, love and self-discipline (2 Timothy 1:7).

*Resilience - Diabetes has helped me be tougher. In high

school, I played (and most importantly, practiced) for a few years under one tough football coach. As a boy whose dad was a functioning alcoholic and whose family was beset with problems, my disciplinary upbringing was terribly inconsistent. Without going into all of the gory details, I will just say that my football coach became a much-needed source of discipline (more narrowing of the gap), but the pancreas just did not cooperate with his player development plan for me—nor with mine.

I loved football, was a determined competitor in the sport, and played until an injury before the start of my junior year did not heal properly for a much longer time than projected. I played through diabetes for those few years previous, and was more resilient as a result. In fact, struggling with the Big D has meant a lifetime of getting knocked down and getting up. Still, my resilience grew by leaps and bounds after I embraced what Jesus went through for me. I started prayerfully getting up with him—repeatedly knocked down, but always getting back up!

We are hard pressed on every side, but not crushed; perplexed, but not in despair; persecuted, but not abandoned; struck down, but not destroyed. We always carry around in our body the death of Jesus, so that the life of Jesus may also be revealed in our body (2 Corinthians 4:8-10).

*Humility - Diabetes has definitely helped me gain humility. If you've been living with either type for any length of time, you probably know what I mean. If you don't, surely you will soon. Our humility grows when we accept the fact that we can't be successful strugglers without lots of help. My hard-learned objective is to embrace my weakness and allow diabetes to be part of the constructive process of making me the person I was made to be—easily said, right?

In facing diabetes, what you bring to the table generally won't be adequate. That is not all bad because God's constructive process requires humility. If you let it, diabetes will be a great tool in God's building of you! Sometimes, I have confused myself about humility, thinking of it as a loss of self-esteem. The great Christian writer, C.S. Lewis said, *Humility is not thinking less of yourself, it's thinking of yourself less.* I like that, and I need to grow in it, for sure. Diabetes deserves attention, but it does not define me. It is part of a constructive process!

He called a little child to him, and placed the child among them. And he said: "Truly I tell you, unless you change and become like little children, you will never enter the kingdom of heaven. Therefore, whoever takes the lowly position of this child is the greatest in the kingdom of heaven (Matthew 18:2-4).

I am convinced that all of the challenges we face are useful. I'm not saying that I always "feel" that way, but in the long run, I always end up facing him and believing it by faith. I trust God when he tells me that diabetes is one part of a constructive struggle. "Facing him" is the focal key I seek.

And we know that in all things God works for the good of those who love him (Romans 8:28).

So we fix our eyes not on what is seen, but on what is unseen, since what is seen is temporary, but what is unseen is eternal (2 Corinthians 4:18).

10

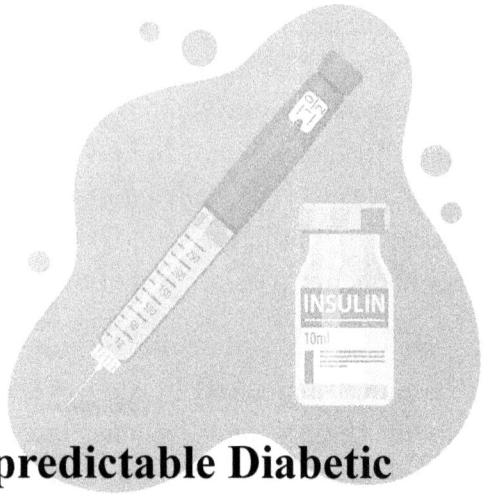

The Unpredictable Diabetic

Curve Balls—

Has anyone ever told you that diabetic calculations are sometimes just attempts to get into the ballpark of accuracy? I think that point has been made in this book, but what about encountering curve balls once you get in the ballpark? I have definitely experienced this.

Yes, I can be looking for a fastball because—for one thing—I may think the variable of insulin dosage (or, for you type 2s, whatever injection or oral medication) is correctly set per a CGM read of my glucose level. I may feel the same for those diet and exercise variables, but my resulting glucose level still does not make a lick of sense.

The expected fastball somehow became the unexpected curve ball, and, whiff! I swing and miss the ball by a foot. "Strike three, you're out!" I can see it now. I look at the umpire with my scowl face, not because his call is wrong, but because he yelled it so loud! I slowly turn, hang my diabetic head, and dejectedly drag my diabetic bat back to the diabetic dugout, only to find myself being gleefully received at the opponent's dugout! Somehow, I got turned around. Talk about adding insult to injury!

Hey, there is even a subset of diabetics who might as well

be called "the unpredictables." (How about forming a baseball team by that name?) This simple statement comes from the Cleveland Clinic, another reliable medical source: *People with brittle Diabetes experience sudden and frequent changes in blood glucose levels for no obvious reason. The swings lead to hypoglycemia or hyperglycemia.*

I was never called an "unpredictable", but I was once told I had a "brittle" form of diabetes by a very qualified physician. He used the term only once, but I could see the grounds he used for it. I think he regretted using it because it's not exactly morale boosting to think of yourself as "brittle"! I was in my thirties and had faced my share of doctors lecturing me on how I needed more self-control in terms of diet and exercise. I was not a really bad diabetic, but I wasn't a really good one either.

I think this pretty good doctor was frustrated with me. No subsequent doctor used the term, but there is a kernel of truth in the application for all of us because unpredictables do indeed exist for diabetics, even for the more regulated ones. Our diabetes does not have to be brittle to be at least somewhat unpredictable. Maybe mine is more so than yours—maybe not.

I do experience times when my glucose levels do not match the known variables at all. It may be higher than I would think it should be considering those variables, and it may be lower. I may have had the amount of exercise and nourishment that would normally make me think my glucose levels should drop, but it rises instead. An expected higher level may sometimes turn out lower than expected. It isn't something that occurs daily, just enough for me to say struggling successfully is made more challenging by unpredictability and inexactitude. The main question, brittle or not, is how do we adjust so the long run effects are minimized.

If you use a continuous glucose monitor like me, you know it can be very accurate. You also know, by periodic calibrations using blood test strips, that it can be off enough to deceive you into taking too much or too little insulin. That difference may be only one or two units of insulin or other measurement of whatever therapeutic you use, but it's still a big deal. Again, it's not frequent for me, but is definitely a reinforcement for occasional calibrations

Regardless of my unpredictables, I have become what I prefer think of as a successful struggler, something I see as a result of God's grace—though at one time I would not have given even a nod to God. If a doctor calls you brittle, or you strike out due to unpredictables, don't drag your bat! Hoist it up on your shoulder, and raise up that chin! <u>Keep your head up and walk with determination to the dugout. You can talk it over with your coach, be a learner, and improve. Strikeouts are bound to come, but if your head is up, at least you'll go to the right dugout</u>!

The best batters in the major leagues only get a hit every three times at bat, and you can do much better with your glucose. Do you know that a specific insulin dose will not necessarily have the same glucose effect for all of us? That's true regardless of diet and exercise variables! Differences can relate to metabolic rates and other things we don't even need to think about.

Suffice to say that our bodies are not replicated machines. God made us to be individuals whose workings are wondrously different. We know that's true by the simplest things, like how a raw onion affects me versus how it affects you. I think we should spare each other the details on that—please!

By the way, if we are comparing notes with another diabetic or with a group, we should question comparisons very carefully. For instance, I told another diabetic that I try to speed walk at least two miles every day. I didn't know if it was one-upmanship or what, but his reply was that he walked further in his neighborhood. When he mentioned the name of his neighborhood, I was familiar with it. It was a flat neighborhood with no hills whereas mine was very hilly.

The Unpredictable Diabetic

Yes, I carefully explained the difference to that guy. Was that one-upmanship? Well, maybe, but the point is that even the variables may sometimes vary, so trust but verify when comparing notes! What someone else does may not be the same, so the result may not predictably be the same for you or me. That does not negate all of the more accurate or positive comparisons.

Here is an article from the Mayo Clinic on still another unpredictable or unexpected aspect of diabetes that isn't often discussed:

What is the dawn phenomenon that some people with diabetes experience? Can anything be done about it?

Answer From M. Regina Castro, M.D.

The dawn phenomenon is an early-morning rise in blood sugar, also called blood glucose, in people with diabetes. The dawn phenomenon leads to high levels of blood sugar, a condition called hyperglycemia. It usually happens between 4 a.m. and 8 a.m.

The cause of the dawn phenomenon isn't clear. Some researchers believe the overnight release of certain hormones that happens naturally increases insulin resistance. That causes blood sugar to rise. The hormones are called counter-regulatory hormones because they have an effect that opposes the effect of insulin. They include growth hormone, cortisol, glucagon and epinephrine.

High blood sugar in the morning may be caused by:

Not getting enough insulin the night before.

Not getting the right dose of diabetes medicine the night before.

Eating a snack with carbohydrates in it at bedtime.

If your blood sugar is consistently higher than it should be in the morning, talk to your health care provider. Your provider may suggest that you check your blood sugar once during the early-morning hours for a few days in a row. Or you might use a continuous glucose monitor to keep track of your blood sugar level as you sleep. That information helps your health care provider confirm if you have the dawn phenomenon or if there could be another reason for high morning blood sugar.

What you can do

To help you prevent or correct high blood sugar in the morning, your health care provider may suggest that you:

- *Avoid carbohydrates at bedtime.*
- *Change your dose of diabetes medicine or insulin.*
- *Switch to a different diabetes medicine.*
- *Change the time when you take your medication or insulin from dinnertime to bedtime.*
- *Use an insulin pump to give you extra insulin during early-morning hours.*

As mentioned before, I experienced the dawn phenomenon. My doctor's suggested splitting of the insulin dosage worked for me. Maybe it will for you, maybe not. Talk to your doctor about the possible "dawn phenomenon" you experience. He or she may not admit it, but I bet you will make a big impression just by using the term! Watch the doctoral facial expression when you say it! If there's no change, hang in. You'll get a rise out of that doctor sometime soon, and something else in this book just might help!

"Calibration" is another impressive-sounding term that you might want to run by your doctor. It sounds downright scientific, right? As I mentioned previously, I do occasional calibrations to ensure the accuracy of my Dexcom G7 CGM. While no longer required (as it was with the G5), I have learned to do this when first installing new units or when having serious accuracy doubts. The latter deserves more attention, but first I want to answer a question that might be nagging you, especially if you're like me and tend to nitpick occasionally.

Why would I include this calibration stuff in a chapter titled, "The Unpredictable Diabetic"? Think of it this way: CGMs are designed to make our predictions more accurate, so in a way, significantly inaccurate CGM results make us less predictable diabetics, i.e. more unpredictable! I know it sounds like a stretch to fit calibrating into this chapter. That's because it is a stretch, but it needs to go somewhere!

Regardless of the stretch, calibrations—and especially those prompted by "serious accuracy doubts"—deserve attention. For me, serious accuracy doubts usually occur after feelings and circumstances are far out of touch with CGM readings (like feeling good a few hours after a light meal and moderate exercise versus a high glucose reading, etc.). In my experience, different forms of this might occur three or four times every month. Since the sensor portion of the G7 currently must be changed after ten days plus a 12-hour grace period, I choose to go ahead and calibrate each time I change the sensor. Therefore, I would say that I calibrate my G7 an average of five times a month, including accuracy doubt calibrations. My calibrations are done by obtaining a drop of blood (ouch!) and applying it to a strip inserted into a glucometer in order to obtain a glucose reading that may be entered into my iPhone CGM app in order to verify CGM results or adjust results for accuracy.

Ensuring that my CGM glucose readings are pretty accurate is important enough to me to do these calibrations. It means that my diet, exercise, and insulin adjustments are going to be on the mark more consistently. I will be a more predictable diabetic. Also, my fingers are definitely not the pin cushions they used to be prior to CGMs, and I'm downright thankful for that! As usual, I must say that you are not me (yes, you know this), so be sure you <u>discuss the calibration business with those paying attention, knowing something, and caring</u>—especially your good doctor!

Again, I say that we all struggle. What's easy about it? The variables of diet, exercise, and insulin are inconsistent and not necessarily measurable and controllable to the same degree at any given time. Something as important as metabolic rates varies for each of us. Your body is not like mine. If your metabolic rate makes it easier for you, or is more consistent than mine, great! If mine is better for the Big D, please don't hold it against me. It's true, and any doctor who does not readily agree that I will struggle, that there are unpredictables, and that treatment is not always an exact science is not one I want doctoring my diabetes.

I don't expect a doctor to make a big deal about metabolisms because that's not something he, she, or we can change for improvement of our diabetes management. The only reason I'm talking about metabolism here is to emphasize again that the variables are not 100% controllable.

Some other things are inconsistent besides our bodies: our attitudes and inclinations! I might just have a positive attitude that works better for the struggle than yours or vice-versa. My inclinations (as natural to me or as developed over time) may work better with diabetes. Yours might fit better than mine. I might be more disciplined, so maybe better prepared for the struggle, or you might be more disciplined than me. I will say it again in different words (better or not): Nothing about diabetes or about us as individuals insulates us from the struggle. Each of us just needs to grow in our ability to struggle well.

Still another unpredictable aspect of diabetes is that complications may very well be caused, exacerbated, or sped up development-wise by either type. These are the things we don't want to talk about or even think about. Isn't it enough to think about diabetes itself? Well, it's true that paying enough attention to our diabetes increases our odds of never having to deal with complications or, at least, dealing with them less, maybe later rather than sooner. However, many of us already have complications, and others need to understand just enough to pick up on signs and take proactive measures. Also, let's be real. It it would not be smart to ignore possibilities that have such enormous implications for our lives and for those who care about us.

If you think I'm stretching again to get this subject matter in the chapter, you are right again! If nothing else, you should feel reinforced in your ability to spot stretches! Now, surely you see that complications will very likely be sooner and more harmful the less you tend to your diabetes, but can you now, or could you before complications, predict or have predicted when or how bad complications will or would be? No? Then, complications for us are … (drum roll)… unpredictable! How'd I do?

No matter the diabetes type, I understand that recent research has shown the buildup of lows in terms of glucose can be negatives in terms of complicating co-morbidities such as cardio conditions, and long-term negatives from continuing highs are well established. Don't worry—I'm not going to drone on about this. In fact, I'll let the Mayo Clinic do the talking, but I'll close it out with some up talk because complications are not all powerful!

Complications -

Long-term complications of diabetes develop gradually. The longer you have diabetes — and the less controlled your blood sugar — the higher the risk of complications. Eventually, diabetes complications may be disabling or even life-threatening. In fact, prediabetes can lead to type 2 diabetes. Possible complications include:

- *Heart and blood vessel (cardiovascular) disease. Diabetes majorly increases the risk of many heart problems. These can include coronary artery disease with chest pain (angina), heart attack, stroke and narrowing of arteries (atherosclerosis). If you have diabetes, you're more likely to have heart disease or stroke.*

- *Nerve damage from diabetes (diabetic neuropathy). Too much sugar can injure the walls of the tiny blood vessels (capillaries) that nourish the nerves, especially in the legs. This can cause tingling, numbness, burning or pain that usually begins at the tips of the toes or fingers and gradually spreads upward. Damage to the nerves related to digestion can cause problems with nausea, vomiting, diarrhea or constipation. For men, it may lead to erectile dysfunction.*

- *Kidney damage from diabetes (diabetic nephropathy). The kidneys hold millions of tiny blood vessel clusters (glomeruli) that filter waste from the blood. Diabetes can damage this delicate filtering system.*

- *Eye damage from diabetes (diabetic retinopathy). Diabetes can damage the blood vessels of the eye. This could lead to blindness.*

- *Foot damage. Nerve damage in the feet or poor blood flow to the feet increases the risk of many foot complications.*

- *Skin and mouth conditions. Diabetes may leave you more prone to skin problems, including bacterial and fungal infections.*

- *Hearing impairment. Hearing problems are more common in people with diabetes.*

- *Alzheimer's disease. Type 2 diabetes may increase the risk of dementia, such as Alzheimer's disease.*

- *Depression related to diabetes. Depression symptoms are common in people with type 1 and type 2 diabetes.*

Complications of gestational diabetes

Most women who have gestational diabetes deliver healthy babies. However, untreated or uncontrolled blood sugar levels can cause problems for you and your baby.

Complications in your baby can be caused by gestational diabetes, including:

- *Excess growth. Extra glucose can cross the placenta. Extra glucose triggers the baby's pancreas to make extra insulin. This can cause your baby to grow too large. It can lead to a difficult birth and sometimes the need for a C-section.*

- *Low blood sugar. Sometimes babies of mothers with gestational diabetes develop low blood sugar (hypoglycemia) shortly after birth. This is because their own insulin production is high.*

- *Type 2 diabetes later in life. Babies of mothers who have gestational diabetes have a higher risk of developing obesity and type 2 diabetes later in life.*

- *Death. Untreated gestational diabetes can lead to a baby's death either before or shortly after birth.*

- *Complications in the mother also can be caused by gestational diabetes, including:*

- *Preeclampsia. Symptoms of this condition include high blood pressure, too much protein in the urine, and swelling in the legs and feet.*

- *Gestational diabetes. If you had gestational diabetes in one pregnancy, you're more likely to have it again with the next pregnancy.*

Okay, I have some of this, but not as bad as it could be, considering. Still, I say whew! Mayo can drone on, and you might be like me sometimes after hearing or reading stuff like this: I get it! Enough already! Couldn't you just spare me all of that Debbie Downer or Norman Negative talk?

For me, a guy with type 1 diabetes for many years, sometimes I think I've heard it all. Hey, I admit that there are times when I think I know more than my doctor. As far as bad possibilities go, you don't need to lecture me! Usually, when I get pumped up like that, one of two things happen to change my thinking. Either something comes up to expose my ignorance, or I pray about it and find myself looking up at Jesus hanging on the cross for me. I'm not there. I'm here. What do I know? Complications? Ha!

My business, in work and in my life as a Christian, is glorifying God and caring about people. I have learned that God created each one of us to be the unique person he intends for us to be and to do what he wants us to do. Even within his plan and will, there is plenty of room for our unpredictables. Nothing is unpredictable or unmanageable for him!

I have told you these things, so that in me you may have peace. In this world you will have trouble. But take heart! I have overcome the world (John 16:33).

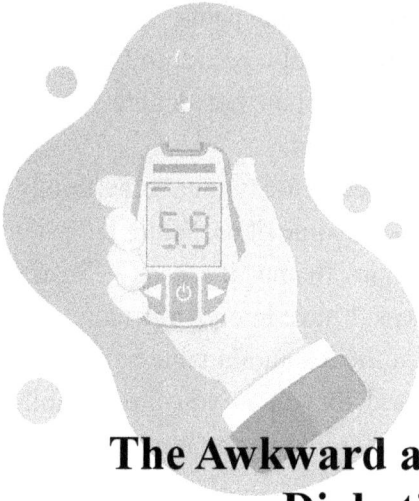

11

The Awkward and/or Scared Diabetic

Now, for you who might lack appreciation for diabetic treatment advances, understand that when I was in college, the home method for testing glucose was filling much of a test tube with your urine, dropping a pill into it, gently swirling the tube around, and waiting to see the liquid's color changed in a way that indicated a very rough range of glucose—pretty primitive, right? It was also just plain awkward, even AWKWARD! (All caps and no cap versions are used herein because sometimes it's big-time to us and sometimes just a little awkward.)

Hey, it's all relative. Back in the earliest days of discovery, the way a doctor knew you had this malady, named or not, was by tasting your sugary urine. Later, when it was discovered that ants would swarm sugar-laden urine and not normal urine, that became the preferred test. I wonder why. Seriously, my guess is that those doctors loved ants!

Anyway, back in the mid-sixties, most of us couldn't even do the pill-in-urine test regularly due to awkwardness. Not only that, but the results were within such a broad range that adjusting insulin, exercise, and diet accordingly was pretty much a joke— not the funny kind, you understand! Adjustments or plan changes based on glucose readings/trends, were way more difficult. It mostly meant flying by the seat of your pants. Think about it. Could you do this urine test in a public restroom? Like I said, AWKWARD! In fact, it was just plain not doable for me. If anyone ever did it, I never knew them.

We diabetics have it a lot better today, but some things are still awkward or AWKWARD for some of us. While I don't want to dwell on the public restroom theme, it's pretty illustrative when it comes to awkwardness. I have known a person who did not hesitate to inject insulin at the restaurant table before dining. I say more power to him and to you if you are uninhibited enough to do that. I am not. Just thinking about it makes me feel awkward.

Before I go too far in expressing admiration for uninhibited diabetics, it must be said that the shot-at-the-table guy also injected right through his shirt! I'm thinking and hoping he's really rare in that regard. Surely, most doctors would frown on the practice. There have to be some healthy inhibitions!

For a long time, when eating out, I took my fast-acting, pre-meal insulin injection in restaurant restrooms, generally in a stall when the room was not a onesie. In recent times, I have found that to be even more AWKWARD because I have developed a neurological condition called focal dystonia in which some manual tasks become difficult due to the fine touch required— writing being an example. Golfers with this condition are often said to have the "yips" when putting. Some famous guitarists have had their careers cut short due to the condition. At any rate, it makes it even more challenging to self-inject insulin in a public restroom so I now prefer to excuse myself to go to the car for a few minutes.

It's an individual deal, but any number of personal things can make any person, diabetic or not, feel awkward. It only deserves mention in the current context because it is among several often unspoken diabetic realities that affect our choices relating to self-regulation.

The Awkward and/or Scared Diabetic

Are you willing to take an injection while sitting at a restaurant table with friends? What about that when it's a lunch business meeting? Do you prefer taking your injection in the public restroom or the car? Some restrooms are more convenient than others, right? Why, I'll have you know that there are some restrooms for men without enclosed stalls—gasp! Okay, I'm reminding myself that what makes me gasp might not phase you at all. Still, I'm reasonably confident that at least a few reading this do relate.

Be aware that even stalls don't always provide perfect privacy. However, over a good many years, I only had one rude stall interruption when taking an injection. It was at Disney World on a crowded day when a perturbed man shouted, "What are you doing in there? You're not even sitting down!" He obviously could see that my feet were not in the proper position for long-term throne occupation. I guess he had a pressing need. My gentle response was to shout back, "I'm taking an injection! Give me a break, okay?" It is so funny to me now, but let's just say that there were two unhappy campers in Mickey's bathroom that day.

As for the car, I have learned that there is no shame in asking for a friend's key if we came in his or her car. At times, when the restroom is a onesie or set up conveniently, it's a no-brainer location for me to take an injection, but when that's not the case, to the car I go!

By the way, since order wait times vary as does the timing of relatively low glucose readings showing up on my CGM, I sometimes do not take my injection until there is reason to believe food is imminent or, sometimes, even until it arrives. Who wants a low to go lower or a hypo to go hypoer (newly coined term)? There is good reason for calling pre-meal insulin "fast-acting" (bolus)! Of course, a glucose pill, candy, sugared drink or juice is the good old go-to if need be! Also, a waiter or waitress will be glad to bring you juice or a coke if needed.

I do understand how some may prefer waiting to inject until after a meal, but I have always found it better pre-meal in terms of timing the effective offset, and a low glucose reading is the only thing that would cause me to forego the injection until post-meal. Of course, other options are skipping that meal, eating sparingly, or waiting for leftovers—"Are you going to eat that?"

One more by-the-way: For a long time, my regular practice has been to inject long-acting insulin in the belly region and fast-acting in the thighs. The reasoning is purely a matter of timing since a thigh or arm injection will act quicker than a stomach or butt injection. I'm good with people using all four sites, but have found administration in the arm or butt personally challenging. Thus, as long as I'm not experiencing atrophy, bruising, etc., I'll stick with my go-tos on this. I hope this transparent description of alternate site usage has not been too AWKWARD for you to read! (If I said "derriere" would everybody understand without googling?)

There is no way to delve into all of the diabetic manifestations of awkwardness. Not only would it require more space than I'm able to provide here, but, again, what is awkward for me may not be awkward for you. Individualized awkwardness is so common that anybody could write a book about that alone, but who wants to be that author? If you're the one, go for it! Speaking of the subject of awkwardness in general, I don't think it deserves a lot of attention. The same is true for diabetic awkwardness unless it is bad enough to keep us from doing what is best for our health. I do believe that happens.

For instance, if my concern keeps me from taking an injection in a timely way before a meal, or worse, taking it at all before eating a meal when my glucose is high, awkward is indeed AWKWARD! In that case, it isn't necessarily necessary that I eradicate the concern. It may well be that I just need to change my response to it—find a way to adapt. In the example, the car generally has become that adaptation for me.

The Awkward and/or Scared Diabetic

If you need help adapting, or if you think your AWKWARDNESS is overblown to the point of anxiety that bogs you down or keeps you from doing what is best, let somebody in on it. Sometimes, a little counseling may be appropriate. As a former counselor, I can tell you that there are those who can be goal oriented and very practical—often short term too. Some of them are Christians using Biblical foundations. A church often can help you connect. One way or another, let somebody in on it who can help.

Now, let's transition from "awkward" to "scared" because we may well be a little of both at times. You understand that, just as we can be part-time deniers but not "Fredish", we can be awkward just sometimes and the same for scared. In fact, a little of both is not bad and can be useful. If you never feel awkward, God bless those around you! We can also use a little fear for reasonable caution purposes, remembering the illustration of a little boy touching a hot stove—you know, healthy fear!

Material quoted from healthline.com previously emphasized emotional or mood effects from extreme glucose levels. This quote from the Mayo Clinic includes more on physical symptoms:

Hypoglycemia needs immediate treatment when blood sugar levels are low. For many people, a fasting blood sugar of 70 milligrams per deciliter (mg/dL), or 3.9 millimoles per liter (mmol/L), or below should serve as an alert for hypoglycemia. But your numbers might be different. Ask your doctor.

If blood sugar levels become too low, signs and symptoms can include:

- *An irregular or fast heartbeat*
- *Fatigue*
- *Pale skin*
- *Shakiness*
- *Anxiety*

- *Sweating*
- *Hunger*
- *Irritability*
- *Tingling or numbness of the lips, tongue or cheek*
- *As hypoglycemia worsens, signs and symptoms can include:*
- *Confusion, abnormal behavior or both, such as the inability to complete routine tasks*
- *Visual disturbances, such as blurred vision*
- *Seizures*
- *Loss of consciousness*

Hypoglycemia potentials are important! Along these lines, I have had some pretty scary instances as a diabetic. My first job out of college included one full day of every work week based at a hospital about forty miles away. I was acting as liaison for an outpatient center where patients would receive aftercare services upon discharge from the hospital. After a busy hospital visit day, I walked to my car in an isolated parking spot.

Nearing the car, I started feeling weak. I sat in the driver's seat, and was sweating profusely by then, but it was not a hot day. I recognized the symptoms of hypoglycemia, but had forgotten my usual candy for such occasions. I tried to open the car door, but found myself losing muscle control. I actually began thrashing around in the car, unable to call for help. Within a few minutes, I was virtually immobilized and barely holding on to consciousness.

Then, he came. A man opened the car door. All I could remember later was this very tall man asking if I needed help. I muttered something like "candy" or "sugar". The man left and returned with the largest peppermint stick I had ever seen! I quickly devoured the whole thing, regaining muscle control and my wits.

I looked around, but the man was gone. After stopping for

food reinforcements on the way home, you can believe that I determined to keep fast-acting sugary snacks available, not just in my pocket, but in the car as well!

After the incident, despite my best efforts, I never found that good Samaritan. A self-proclaimed atheist then, I was not fazed by my wife's insistence that the man was an angel. Today, I would not put that past God—not at all! In fact, I hereby assert a retroactive claim for my angel! Given the availability of the CGM today, someone could say it is unlikely to happen again. I say that the odds are better, but CGMs do not rule. I still have bad lows—rare, but I have them. Sometimes, you just cannot be sure about the glucose drop rate.

The parking lot incident was a good fear lesson for me. <u>Have a healthy fear of the scary lows, certainly enough to never neglect your anti-hypo supply stock, in your pocket, purse, car, etc.</u>

One more fear-reinforcing example might be helpful. Once, I was driving down the busiest four-lane of a pretty big city when that devil hypoglycemia caught up to me pronto. I was not as hypo sensitive or perceptive then, and there was no good way to really track glucose levels and trends proactively—certainly not accurately in real time. I did the urine "test' a couple of times a day or sometimes only once in those days. The hypo hit me quick while driving. I lost muscle control. The car swerved in a semi-circle and came to a stop crossways in the middle of this busy highway with lots of wheels screeching behind. A huge traffic jam followed, compliments of yours truly!

One of the dangerous things about bad hypoglycemia is that it can disorient you. I did not lose consciousness, but you could say I was semiconscious when a man stuck his head inside the open passenger side window to ask if I was okay. As was the case with the parking lot incident, I couldn't say much except the magic word, "sugar". A good bystander gave me a Coke. By the time a police officer opened my car door and addressed me, I was fine.

Later, the state of my residence instituted a law requiring what amounted to an annual doctor's driving permission slip for those with diabetes (no type 2 then, so no need to say type 1). Advice: Don't drive when drinking, drunk, or even close to hypoglycemic! It must be added that the diabetic driving permission law was repealed. I am not sure why that happened. I'm just thankful that measuring glucose levels became much easier and more accurate, making the odds better for all of us on the road!

Thank God for good Samaritans and angels! Now, about being a scared diabetic, I'm again a part-timer—cautious, healthy fear yes, but not to the point of avoiding real life. Sometimes, people live their lives all wrapped up in caution tape. Diabetes deserves attention and a lot of life adjustments, but it does not deserve control of our lives—no way, no how! However, we should have enough healthy fear not to drive hypo! When we err, we should set things up for erring on the side of safety by keeping glucose-raising sustenance near enough to get to it quick and by making any adjustments for the sake of reasonable caution.

Stay with me on this while we talk morbidly. "Co-morbidities" became a popular term during Covid, or at least, many of us picked up on the term then because it was being used so much to describe how having Covid could affect you when you have other serious conditions. No, I do not use the term "morbid", co or otherwise, in everyday conversation or even now and then. Look, it is a yucky term to use—a morbid word, right?

To be honest, I'm using it only because we diabetics better get used to it—get de-sensitized, a fancy word meaning get used to it. Beyond that, I'm issuing this public service announcement: Diabetics have a lot of important components in play besides pancreases and livers. We are like other humans with teeth, feet, and eyes—as well as a lot of unseen internal stuff, organs like lungs and hearts! We are intricate, imperfect physical beings, and with time and wear, things do go wrong. The fact is that all humans live with morbidity potentials.

Then, it's like those dominoes we set on end and lined up

in a winding snake pattern. With a finger tap, the front one falls back, and others behind it go down in consecutive order as each one hits another—except for the last one that has nothing to hit. For many of us, type 1 diabetes is the domino that starts or just speeds up a lot of other nasties (cardio, kidney, etc.). Actually, our first domino may be a gene or antibody. For the majority of type 2s (not all), obesity is the first domino, but it might really be a gene or both. Does it matter? No, so what does matter?

For all of us, lifestyle adjustments may increase the distance between the first and second domino—a preventive strategy. Insulin alone just won't do it. For most type 2s, lifestyle adjustments potentially prevent the first domino of obesity from toppling the second which may well be the big D! Pills and shots alone just won't do it anyway you cut it.

In your case, I feel really optimistic because you have read this much of what's not the easiest book to stomach, with all the lifestyle, transparency, and other challenging talk. You're wanting to gain better control. You've probably already imagined those dominoes so quickly falling in succession and uniformly, but you know that complications in real life are rarely uniform. Now, imagine them in slow motion, some of them anyway. Get the idea?

So, how much fear does all this stuff deserve? Well, it's true that living is a risk. We could opt to live like Howard Hughes who cut himself off from real day-to-day life out of a paralyzing fear, or we can accept the fact that fear is available to be constructive so avoid touching the hot stove, but cook on it!

Fear can indeed be constructive. However, if fear becomes anxiety to the point that it causes us to avoid things in life that are loaded with good potential, we should share our struggle with someone, perhaps a counselor or minister, but certainly someone who wants to help.

This has been a tough chapter. Much of this book has been tough, but you and I can and should take heart! Consider that a lot of things are now much more manageable. Consider all of the treatment advances. Consider that none of them include the cabbage-and-water-only 6-month treatment! Consider that we are so very blessed. Consider the room for improvement in our struggle and the opportunities it presents us to help each other. Over it all, please consider God whose love for us is personal and proven on a cross!

If this book helps you in any way, the credit goes to God. I am praying for your health physically and spiritually. No matter where you stand on your journey, the following words of assurance bear repeating:

Do not be anxious about anything, but in every situation, by prayer and petition, with thanksgiving, present your requests to God. And the peace of God, which transcends all understanding, will guard your hearts and your minds in Christ Jesus (Philippians 4:6-7).

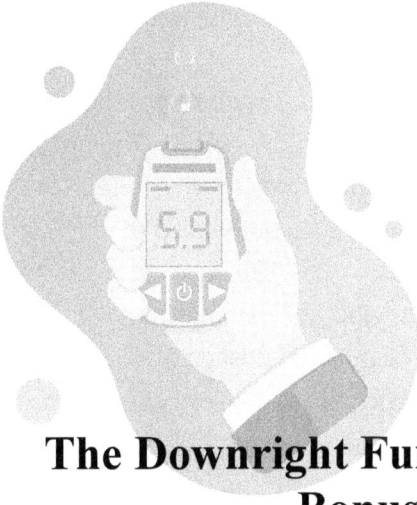

12

The Downright Funny Diabetic—A Bonus!

Just a few weeks before finishing this project, yours truly did something harmful to my efforts toward successful diabetes management. It was the cause of panic in our household. Today, however, I consider it to be an example of how a valuable tool in my diabetes toolbox works.

The tool is a sense of humor. The prerequisite for using it is that a funny thing happens. As such, this incident is something to share with you in closing.

It was just a routine day. My wife was preparing our dinner (or as I used to say, supper). I was preparing to take my two usual evening insulin injections: long-acting Lantus at a set dosage (basal) of 14 and fast-acting Novolog at a variable dosage (bolus) according to the CGM reading and meal content. The bolus (Novolog) dosage was to be 6 on this occasion.

As a creature of habit, I was watching tv news while going through my injection routine. I injected the fast-acting 6 units of Novolog first as usual since my wife had given me the standard 15-minute advance notice before our meal would be ready. Something on the news caught my attention. At that moment, I removed the needle and placed the cap over my Novolog insulin pen. Since I had already removed the cap from my "Lantus" pen,

I just affixed the needle and injected that long-term dosage of 14 units.

Everything seemed routine until I started to put the cap over the "Lantus" pen. It was not the right color—Novolog blue instead of Lantus gray. An accurate term for my thought at that moment would be, "Huh?" I had mistakenly used the fast-acting Novolog pen (blue cap) twice! Now, for you who are math-challenged like me, here is the operable calculation: $6 + 14 = 20$ or approximately 3.3 times the planned dosage of 6! Now, folks, that's not happy calculating because such an insulin overage, if not dealt with promptly, could produce what I'll call nightmarish hypoglycemia! You know that panic adrenalin surge? I had it!

I informed my wife. If the conversation that followed was recorded, it would be well described as a cacophony. I think the Cambridge Dictionary definition applies: *a loud, unpleasant mixture of sounds*. I'm not sure about octaves, but they had to be high flying. The visual would include flailing arms and big eyes. Subsequently, my math was followed by hers, only much faster!

The litany of consumables entering yours truly's mouth thereafter would be impossible to recite. It did not include the kitchen sink. A few things stand out in my memory: glucose pills, some type of snack bar, grape juice, and even syrup—no lemon pie! While my wife shuffled stuff to me, I would periodically blurt out a few things: "I think that's enough." "I'm okay." Still, my CGM low glucose alarm went off. Despite continued shuffling and swallowing, I started feeling weak and a little disoriented.

After further ingesting of Lord-knows-what, I regained my faculties enough to say, "I <u>cannot</u> eat any more!" The only symptom by then was a very upset stomach. Later, my CGM reading told me I was approaching the high point of a scary roller coaster ride. I had gone from one extreme to another so it took an extra dose of insulin to bring my glucose level back down to a reasonable level. In the aftermath, what may be best described as a miserable hangover lasted hours.

The Downright Funny Diabetic — A Bonus!

Sure, nobody was laughing throughout this ordeal. However, my wife and I saw the humor in it the next day. We laughed! Laughter is often retro in that way. I am a funny person as are you! The diabetic in you and me is hilarious if we just open up to it. I said this proactively, before my wife could: "I know. The Home is just down the hill, and I can coast to it!" We often invoke the local nursing home for such times of obliviousness. Laughter is inevitable!

You have your own toolbox. This is my final pitch for you to use the humor tool in there—not limited to, but inclusive of, self-effacement. I challenge you to admit to yourself that you are downright hilarious, *intentionally or not*!

The more important challenge follows the first: Laugh at yourself because you are a downright funny person! Diabetes must be taken seriously, but it also provides a lot of comedy material. If you are a Christian, even the exercise of your faith sometimes provides it.

I could tell some stories about me as a downright funny Christian, but that would take another book. I'm sure my dear wife would be happy to be the co-author, but I'm just not ready to write that one. Maybe the *Downright Funny Christian* book is your calling—or not! God bless!

Now to the King eternal, immortal, invisible, the only God, be honor and glory for ever and ever. Amen (1 Timothy 1:17).